the
newborn
twins
sleep guide

the newborn twins sleep guide

The Nap and Nighttime Sanity Saver

for Your Duo's First Five Months

Natalie Diaz, CLC, CPST,
and Kim West, MSW

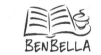

BenBella Books, Inc.
Dallas, TX

The Newborn Twins Sleep Guide copyright © 2024 by KW Media Properties, LLC, and Tired Twin Mom, LLC

BenBella Books, Inc.
10440 N. Central Expressway
Suite 800
Dallas, TX 75231
benbellabooks.com
Send feedback to feedback@benbellabooks.com

BenBella is a federally registered trademark.

Printed in the United States of America
10 9 8 7 6 5 4 3 2 1

Library of Congress Control Number: 2023036380
ISBN 9781637744420 (trade paperback)
ISBN 9781637744437 (electronic)

Editing by Leah Wilson
Copyediting by Jessica Easto
Proofreading by Cape Cod Compositors, Inc. and Lisa Story
Indexing by Amy Murphy
Text design and composition by PerfecType
Cover design by Morgan Carr
Cover image © Adobe Stock / fotoduets
Printed by Lake Book Manufacturing

Special discounts for bulk sales are available. Please contact bulkorders@benbellabooks.com.

This book is dedicated to my one and only, John.
All those sleepless nights with our twinnies
would have been pretty boring without you.
I think it's the only time we were both
appreciative of your insomnia.
Thank you for loving me so fiercely through
this rollercoaster of twin life.
I love you more than all the fish in the ocean
and all the stars in the sky.

—Nat

Contents

Welcome to the Wonderful World of Twins

A stranger on the street asks, "Are they twins?" as they peer into a double stroller.

"Absolutely!" the parent replies.

"Good luck, you'll never sleep again," the stranger says as they walk away.

Ugh! If I had a nickel for every! single! time! someone said this to me when my twins were babies, I wouldn't need to worry about paying for two college tuitions at the same time. I'm not sure where folks get the audacity to make predictions like "double trouble" or the dreaded "get all your rest now, you'll never sleep again." It's jaw dropping. Who says that parents of twins can't sleep? Not ALL parents of twins have kiddos who are up all night, keeping the entire house's eyes open till sunrise.

"How to get my twins to sleep through the night?" is, however, one of the most searched for topics on Twiniversity.com, the world's leading twin parenting resource, which I founded back in 2009. But if we play our cards right, we actually *can* set our family up for restful nights. Raising twins doesn't have to fill you with sleep dread. There are many small ways that you can help your twinnies sleep just a little bit better in the first five months—and together, these can add up to significantly better sleep for everyone!

While it's true that I can't promise you'll never have a night where you'll be up so long that you catch the 5:30 AM news on TV and listen to the anchor's banter about the new sneakers they bought (that's a true story from my own sleepless nights), I *can* tell you that we will set you up for the best chance of sleep-filled nights for both you and your twinnies.

I'm so excited that finally, after more than a decade of friendship, Kim West, The Sleep Lady, and I have paired up to help ensure that *your* twinnies start sleeping through the night as early as possible. Kim has cracked the code on newborn sleep. With over twenty-five years of helping parents around the globe, Kim has learned that raising babies—even newborn twins—doesn't have to be a sleep-deprived nightmare. Her Baby-Led Sleep Shaping and Coaching method is a gentle approach that parents can use to shape sleep at first and then, when developmentally (and temperamentally) appropriate, coach their little ones as they learn to fall asleep and stay asleep on their own.

Kim and I first met when we were both asked to speak together to a group of Southern California moms in Studio City back in 2013. Never in my career have I hit it off with someone so quickly. Despite meeting literally minutes before we went on stage, our lecture went off without a hitch, and although we had some differences of opinion on some things (I was pro–Cry It Out method, and she had her Gentle Sleep Coaching method), we worked together as if we had been doing that speech for years. Afterward, we went to dinner together at Universal Studios, and the rest, as they say, kids . . . is history!

Since then, we've done videos and podcasts together and collaborated on articles. Kim is my go-to sleep pro. She's someone I have the utmost respect for, and her dedication to pediatric sleep is like nothing I've ever seen before. That's why I'm proud to be at her side for our first book collaboration.

By the final pages of this book, you'll feel so much better about the entire sleep process for your twinnies. Kim's decades of working directly with thousands of parents of singletons *and* twinnies has taught her and her team that the sleep techniques we teach are even more effective when parents know *why* they are effective. So, you'll learn not just what to do to help your duo sleep better, sooner, but also all about newborn sleep itself, with age-specific information about how development, feeding, attachment, soothing, and temperament all affect sleep—all customized for twin parents.

Through Twiniversity, I've helped thousands of families across the globe navigate hundreds of issues they've had with their twins. From unique twin pregnancy complications like twin-to-twin transfusion syndrome to common breastfeeding concerns, I work with parents almost daily. My workdays are filled with nothing but twins, and then guess what? I get to go home and deal with my own twins, now eighteen years old and heading off to college. They are magnificent kids, and I'm glad I was chosen to be their mama. But HOLY HECK!!! did they give me a run for my money when it came to sleep. I had one twin, my Baby B, John, who was such a good sleeper. He was like a gift from Mother Nature—payment for all the issues I had during their pregnancy. The other one, however, my Baby A, Anna, may be the sole reason I lost ALL color in my hair after pregnancy. Yup, under this hair dye, I'm completely white! She was an "alert baby" (Kim's term; you'll learn more about this later) and was a constant challenge. Good news, though! She's an amazing young adult with a brilliant head on her shoulders—though, honestly, still a poor sleeper.

My daughter is one of the reasons I'm writing this book with Kim. I assumed that my twins would have similar temperaments and similar sleep patterns and schedules. "HA!" I say to my past self. Having two at the same time doesn't necessarily mean they share anything but a birthday! We'll discuss this in a lot more detail later on, but just know this from these early pages: Your kids are two different tiny people and need to be looked at and treated as such. That goes for sleep as much as anything else.

Over the next few hundred pages, we'll help you build not only the skills to get your duo to sleep but also confidence and trust in the process. When Kim and I would discuss families we were working with, she always gently reminded me that I should never call it "sleep training" like I had been calling it for years. "Nat, it's not sleep training," she'd say. "It's sleep *coaching*. You don't need to *train* a baby to sleep—you have to help them build the skills to self-soothe so they can fall asleep on their own." But no matter what you call it, sleep training or sleep coaching, we are going to get you the same final result: a peaceful night that allows you to enjoy your day—and your twins—even more.

—Nat

chapter one

Please Start Here

Seriously, please start here. We know you're ready to jump into the meat of this book and go right to the chapter based on your twinnies' age, but we need you to learn to walk before you can run. This chapter covers a lot of basics that form the foundation each chapter is built upon. You might find yourself referring back to it often, so grab a pen and start circling parts that you think are important to read again, and perhaps even highlight them for your partner or family members who might be helping you and your twins on your sleep coaching adventure.

Why a Sleep Book That's Made Just for Twin Families?

If you are currently pregnant, you may not know yet how different it is having twins versus a singleton. I'll give you a heads-up: Having two babies demanding your attention at the same time isn't just twice as hard, it's exponentially harder. I'm not saying this to make you nervous; I'm just being real here. It's not "bad" harder, but it is harder. On the flip side, it's exponentially more rewarding as well. Twins are absolutely amazing, and I promise you, speaking to you from the future, while parenting twins is both magical and terrifying, no matter what, it's absolutely extraordinary. I couldn't imagine having just one; that would have been very boring. Many times, I worried I wasn't capable of the task of raising my duo, but now that I have, I'm pretty sure there is LITERALLY nothing I can't handle. Parenting those two gave me confidence beyond my wildest dreams and a feeling of self-fulfillment that I didn't know was possible. You'll have the same, I assure you. You just gotta get through some rough spots—and the first five months will have a few.

What does this have to do with sleep? Well, sleep can be one of those rough spots. But also, sleep for both you and your twins is critical for negotiating the bumps in the road ahead. Consider this book a paving crew designed to make your journey a little smoother.

So why do you need a sleep book *just* for twins? Many sleep books only mention dealing with twins once or twice and very vaguely, which I know from experience can leave you feeling isolated. The world often seems made for singleton babies when you were dealt two. Our book is 100 percent about you and your crew.

Let me break it down a little more . . .

1. Most sleep books discuss the basic challenges of sleep but not the challenge of juggling two same-age sleepers at once.

2. "Sleep when the baby sleeps," common advice, isn't realistic when you have twins because there a good chance one kiddo will be awake when the other is snoozing. Twin parents need to schedule their own sleep when feasible and create some predictability around their twins' sleep as soon as possible.

3. Most sleep books don't discuss the NICU and preterm delivery in as much detail as necessary. These topics play a common role in many twin families' experiences.

4. Most sleep books provide instructions for sleep coaching with two adults. With twins, however, you'll often need three folks to make it work.

Your twins may be very different people. This means different temperaments and different needs. Many families assume that twins will be on the same schedule *all the time*. Not true—you might have two kiddos who are very different (like I did), and you'll need to react to them accordingly. That can mean needing to enact two different approaches to sleep coaching—at the same time (which is where having those three adults can come in handy!). Twins also often reach milestones at different times, which can affect sleep.

In short, supporting your newborn twins in getting to sleep and staying asleep through the night is a lot more complicated. Our advice is tailored specifically to *your* family and sets you up for greater success by taking the unique challenges of twin parenthood into account. Our goal: to fill your sleep toolbox with tricks and tips that you'll apply not only to this set of twins but your next set as well. (Yup, that happens—so be forewarned!)

Why Cry It Out May Be a Waste of Time for Your Twins

Under the traditional sleep training umbrella, you'll find two different methods: the extinction method (also known as Cry It Out) and the graduated extinction method. The extinction method instructs parents to put their baby to bed fully awake and exit the room, allowing them to cry until they figure out how to get themselves to sleep. The idea behind this sleep method is that, by allowing your kiddos to fall asleep on their own, they will learn the process all by themselves. The graduated extinction method is virtually the same but adds in timed intervals where a parent pops into their kiddos' room to soothe or check on them as they are crying or fussing.

The origins of the extinction method go way back to the 1920s, when US psychologist Dr. John Watson proposed the concept of behaviorism, which states that a child is a blank canvas and any behavior they exhibit is caused by external stimuli and not related to their internal thoughts or feelings. He taught parents that the way that they reacted to their baby was what shaped their baby's behavior. In other words, if they don't respond to their baby's crying, the baby will no longer cry and simply go to sleep.

Once upon a time, Cry It Out was the most often used method for getting your twins to sleep. Many families would start around the fourth month, but some would attempt it even sooner. It makes sense: Parents of twins are often more desperate for a good night's sleep because, thanks to that second baby, their daily grind is a lot more challenging. You feel like you're on a constant merry-go-round. Days blend into nights blend into days blend into nights and so on. A solid chunk of sleep (more than four hours) breaks up that ride, and since many twin families don't know that you can set your twinnies up for happier and healthier sleep sooner, they jump right into Cry It Out because they feel they have nothing to lose. But I have a feeling that you're trying to get a jump start and avoid the drama of Cry It Out, since you bought this book. (Thank you, by the way, if I haven't said that already!)

Cry It Out may work for some people, but it ignores several big developmental factors that play a role in a baby's ability to fall asleep:

- The ability to put oneself to sleep, regardless of age, is dependent on the ability to self-soothe. Newborns are not physically or mentally capable of self-soothing just yet.
- Every baby exhibits their own unique temperament that determines how they respond to their external environment—and how difficult they are to soothe.
- A baby can only learn something new when they aren't super stressed and crying their little hearts out. If they get *too* fussy or *too* dysregulated (like when they are hysterically crying), they actually *can't* learn the new skills that would help them self-soothe.

In a nutshell, newborns can't cry it out. It's why most docs don't really recommend it before four months. Babies aren't developmentally ready to put themselves to sleep before that; it happens later on down the line as they mature.

I have to be honest here. For many, many years, I've talked about sleep training and the old-school Cry It Out method in our Twiniversity classes. Remember that story I told you at the beginning of this book, where Kim and I were on a panel discussing sleep? She was the Gentle Sleep Coach and I was the hard-core "shut the door and run for your life" speaker. I'm very proud to say that I've evolved. During the past decade, working with so many families of twins, I've learned that Kim was right. That's why I knew I needed to get this book into your hands today.

Back when my twins were babies, I personally resorted to the antiquated Cry It Out method, and HOLY MOLY GUACAMOLE it was tough—not just on them but on me. I now know that it was challenging not only because of . . . hello . . . insane amounts of crying, but also because there is a bunch of biology behind a new mom's reaction to hearing her baby cry. A gentler sleep coaching method works wonderfully *and* does not make you want to rip your hair out.

Still worried about NOT letting your twins cry it out? A great 2013 research study by Dr. Pamela Douglas found that sleep training during the first six months of your baby's life does not decrease crying (or prevent sleep and behavioral problems) later in childhood. In fact, sometimes the opposite can happen: Crying can *in*crease (and breastfeeding might stop earlier, besides).

OK, so what do we do now? If we can't sleep train for the first six months, how the heck are we going to get enough rest to be productive members of society? FEAR NOT, my friends! We've got some great tips for how to help shape your twinnies' sleep as they learn the ropes of life and gain some amazing new skills that create a foundation for better sleep down the line—plus guidance on helping your baby learn how to sleep in a way that's appropriate for their developmental stage.

The Difference Between Sleep Shaping and Sleep Coaching

Have you ever heard of Baby-Led Sleep Shaping and Coaching before? Odds are no, since our Sleep Queen Kim West invented it. (See, we only rub elbows with the fanciest of folks with singletons here at Twiniversity. *Ooh la la!*)

Let's take a closer look at these two terms—sleep shaping and sleep coaching—and what they mean.

Sleep shaping is the process of supporting sleep with a parent's or caregiver's help and a healthy sleep environment and practices. It is the approach we recommend for the first three to five months of your newborn twins' lives.

Sleep shaping involves creating safe and healthy sleep-friendly space (dark room, white noise, proper temperature). It also includes regulating your twins' morning wake times and night bedtimes, and a pre-bed routine to let your twins know what to expect next, so they can take an express trip to sleepy town! Sleep shaping basically sets the stage for learning to sleep independently when your twins are developmentally ready.

Sleep coaching is the process of supporting your twins as they learn to put themselves to sleep once they reach a developmentally appropriate age. Like a coach in your favorite sport, you can teach, direct, and support them. But as you know, a coach doesn't *play* the game, and it's the same with sleep coaching: You can't learn to sleep *for* your twins. You are simply helping those twinnies of yours learn the ropes and perfect their own sleep skills.

Sleep coaching involves continuing to support your twins each night as they learn self-soothing techniques and practice putting themselves to sleep. Slowly, you'll do less and less as they eventually do more and more. It also includes tailoring your sleep coaching plan to match your twins' unique temperaments.

Sleep shaping sets the foundation so that you can gently and effectively sleep coach when your twins are ready. Think of it this way: Sleep shaping is the equivalent of stretching before a run, and sleep coaching is training to complete that first big marathon. The training will go smoother if they stretch beforehand. Sleep shaping and sleep coaching work together to make your babies stronger runners . . . I mean sleepers . . . ugh, you know what I mean.

What's Self-Regulation and Why It Matters

You'll hear a lot of talk in this book about your twinnies learning how to self-regulate. Self-regulation is a baby's ability to filter out stimuli and manage their behavior, emotions, and reactions in response to their surrounding environment—for example, by signaling that they are hungry, reacting to a loud person or someone who is too close, or looking for their twinnie if they are feeling lonely. When it comes to falling sleep, learning self-regulation is crucial. It's the key to unlocking the door to all of you getting more rest.

Life in the FAST Lane!

All right, gaggle of parents, you're saying to yourself, "Nat come on, get to the good part, I'm freaking exhausted." I hear you, I do, but sleep is just ONE aspect of your newborn twins' lives. You want to sleep, they want to eat, and you both need to snuggle. So just addressing sleep at this age isn't enough! Feeding, Attachment,

Soothing, and Temperament (FAST) all affect your twinnies' sleep, and that sleep affects you. That's why, in each month, we'll look at all four of these factors.

Let's break it down (insert beatboxing noises here).

Feeding

If your twinnies aren't eating well, I'd wager they aren't sleeping well, either. When it comes to feeding, just following the recommended guidelines laid out by your doc for each age can do wonders to support daytime and nighttime sleep. Think about this: Can you go to sleep hungry? Can you eat when you're super sleepy? See what I mean? They each have an impact on the other. (OK, for the record, I can pretty much always eat, no matter how tired I am, but that's the Italian blood in me speaking. Actually, I'm going to grab a snack right now. Hang on. BRB.)

Attachment

I'm gonna throw on my nerd glasses for a second. (Ahem.) German psychoanalyst Erik Erikson found that humans go through eight stages of psychosocial development throughout their life. During the first eighteen months, his theory says, babies are learning about trust. (Awww!) Your twins are learning to trust that, when they call out for you to help them, you'll be there, and this trust is the foundation for what psychologists call attachment: the lasting bond between a parent and a child based on the child's trust that their needs—like being fed and cared for—will be provided for. (Removes nerd glasses.)

Attachment is what creates that secure bond with your twins. It not only provides a feeling of safety and security for them but also helps you, as a parent, understand your kiddos' cues—which is the basis of learning how best to soothe them.

Soothing

Soothing is how you help your duo become regulated when they are dysregulated—when they are crying and unhappy and (because they are still just babies) unable to manage their emotions.

When it comes to soothing, one of the biggest questions we hear is this: "Am I creating bad habits by responding to my twins too much?" At this age, the answer is a resounding *nope*! Your job as a parent of newborns is to help your babies get to a soothed state so that they know what it feels like. Once they understand what the "all is well" state is like, they'll want to get back there. Your babies get uncomfortable and cry, you soothe them, and they feel better—repeat over and over again. As they grow older, they will start to develop self-soothing skills (say that three times fast!) that will help them get there on their own, but in the meantime, soothing them is up to those who are caring for them.

Congratulations on Your Promotion! It's Time to SOAR

 Oh, I forgot to tell you, you just got promoted at your parenting twins job. In addition to everything else you have to do, now you also have to play baby detective. While yes, that totally sounds like a new show on Netflix (*Baby Detective*, episode 1: "The Case of the Missing Binkies"), being a new baby detective is really about gathering clues to better decipher your twins' needs and how best to meet them—a crucial part of attachment and soothing that will ultimately play a big role in sleep shaping and coaching.

Just because you now have twins doesn't mean you are magically able to understand them. That's a myth I'd like to debunk right here and now. Please don't feel like you're a bad parent because you don't instantly understand what your twins want the moment they are born. You need to get to know them and their unique communication styles, just like they are learning yours.

So, how do you become a master baby detective? By learning to SOAR.

SOAR is an acronym Kim created that stands for **S**top, **O**bserve, **A**ssess, and **R**espond, and it's designed to help you figure out what might be causing your babies' fussiness or crying. Keeping this tiny acronym top of mind will give you a gentle reminder of the process that you should follow to solve the mystery that is your twins! It gives you concrete steps to take when you feel at a loss for how to respond to your babies. Plus, it not only helps at the moment but also builds your understanding of their baby language so that you are more prepared the next time you are trying to figure out why they might be cranky.

Here's how to SOAR, step-by-step:

Stop . . . take a breath and don't react out of fear or frustration.

Observe . . . what your baby or babies are doing. Pay attention to the sounds they are making, the way they are moving, and the surroundings they are in. Are they giving you any signals? Are their arms and legs pulled in? Are they looking away? What are they doing with their bodies and their faces? Are their diapers full? Are they extra warm or extra cool?

Assess . . . the current situation. What is their current environment like? What has occurred within the recent past that could be making them squirmy? Were there visitors? New smells? Loud noises? How do the signals they're giving off correlate with their behavior, environment, and/or activities over the last few hours? You will eventually learn cues that your kids may exhibit related to hunger, soothing needs, sleepiness, and their individual temperament, both from this book and from observing your baby over time.

Respond . . . once you've determined the likely best action to meet your kiddos' needs. You might soothe them, quiet the environment, snuggle them, feed them, or assist them in going to sleep for a nap or the night.

So, what are you going to say in your head when your babies look like they just bought a ticket on the Hot Mess Express? "SOAR." Correct! *Stop. Observe. Assess. Respond.*

See, you're getting the hang of this! That was a well-deserved promotion. You're a great parent, and your twinnies are lucky that they have you.

Temperament

Understanding your babies' temperaments is key to understanding their unique sleep patterns and abilities. Different temperaments respond differently to various soothing, sleep shaping, and sleep coaching techniques. This is one of the most unique challenges with twins. "Because of the extraordinary complexity of the human brain, which ensures its individuality, no two people are ever alike—not even identical twins," says Joan Friedman, one of the premier twin psychology experts in the world.

Maybe one twin is typically very happy while the other is typically super fussy. Perhaps you have one who is super passive while their twin is much more alert and active. It happens. This isn't something that can be predicted. One of your first jobs as a new parent is to learn to work with your babies' temperaments and not in opposition. Yes, this can be a challenge and will make your head spin for a minute or two, but you'll find that, in no time at all, you'll understand all their many moods. And you will not only come to understand them but also predict said moods based on prior experiences. This will come in handy as you sleep shape and ultimately create the sleep coaching plan that is the best match for all of you.

Looking Out for #1 . . . YOU!

OK, hear me out. You need to pay attention to yourself. I want to repeat this over and over again because I can't stress enough the importance of taking care of YOU!

Each month Twiniversity has a virtual meeting (find out how to join us at Twiniversity.com/membership) that includes an open discussion about twin life, where the moms and dads in attendance are free to discuss any and all topics that are causing them stress. As a group, we work on different strategies that can make their twin life better.

Time after time after time, we have to remind parents that they need to put their own oxygen mask on first before assisting others, just like they say at the start of each plane ride you take.

Month after month we see how twin parents are on the verge of collapse due to exhaustion, frustration, and confusion. The first thing I usually ask is, "When was the last time you left the house?" It sounds like such a silly question, but more often than not, especially if their kids are under four months old, they are stumped.

I warn you, if you do not take care of yourself, you will pay the price. Here are some things that may happen if you neglect yourself while parenting twins:

- You won't be able to fully enjoy the amazing children you've made and may even start to resent them.
- You'll feel like an extra in a zombie movie, going through the paces of your day without having much memory of it—meaning you'll forget

some super sweet memories because your brain is too exhausted to hold on to them. This is the saddest one for me because I fell into this category a lot.

- You'll start to feel like the Tin Man from *The Wizard of Oz*: Your body will start to get achy because it's crying out for you to rest.
- You'll lose yourself in parenthood and forget that you are an amazing person outside your twinnie world and capable of almost anything.
- Your self-esteem will take a hit. Exhaustion can make it hard to do even the simplest things correctly, which can make it feel like the world is caving in on you.
- Your stress will become your family's stress, and your family's stress will become your twinnies' stress. No one needs stressed twinnies.
- You may lose patience and not be as responsive as you want to be toward your twins.
- If you are breastfeeding, your milk production may suffer. If you aren't taking care of yourself and being very thoughtful about your supply, you could jeopardize how much you produce.
- You won't have the energy to support your partner and become a united front as you prepare to sleep coach your duo.

I can seriously go on for days here. I'm not kidding. I regularly watch new twin parents break down in tears. It's why I'm so frustrated teleportation hasn't been invented yet, and I can't just zap myself into their homes and beg them to go take a nap while I take care of their kiddos. When I'm working with a client in person, helping them with lactation, once we've established a trusting rapport, I often throw them out to go take a walk around the block and get their mind back on track. It typically works like a charm.

Since I can't get to you when you might need it, we'll discuss bits of self-care throughout this book. For now, though, keep it top of mind that you need to take care of YOU, too!

So, Where and How Do I Start?

Although this book is organized by age, we need to talk about the twin elephants in the room: prematurity and adjusted age. These two factors play a significant role in how you'll follow the guidance in this book. All of our monthly recommendations are based on your twins' gestational age, and if your kids were born early, you may need to stick with the steps in the first months until you feel they are caught up.

Please keep in mind that there is a lot of variability in the development of all babies in the first five months, premature or not. We share the milestones in order, but your twins might reach them earlier or later (and at different times from one another). Remember, it's not a race! We encourage you to trust your gut and get help from your pediatrician if you have concerns.

In other words, if your twins were premature, you can still follow the advice in this book, but you may be on a different timeline. You'll just use your babies' adjusted age. To figure out their adjusted age, take your twins' actual age in weeks and subtract the number of weeks they were preterm. For example, if your babies are a week shy of three months old but were born seven weeks early, follow the recommendations for one-month-old twinnies regarding Gentle Sleep Coaching (11 weeks – 7 weeks = 4 weeks old). This isn't true for all babies—some parents of twins rarely give adjusted age a second thought—but here, for this book, we think you should seriously consider it as a factor when following our sleep shaping and especially sleep coaching recommendations.

All in all, though, don't get too stressed about adjusted age versus gestational age. As a mom of preemie twins myself (thirty-four-weekers in the house), I assure you that it's common in our multiple-birth world to deliver early.

Getting You and Your Duo to Sleep

The process we offer in this book *will* work to get your twinnies to sleep. Yes, I know you have twins. Yes, I know that, especially if you are dealing with your twins solo, it's going to be a rougher go than it is for singleton parents (story of our lives, am I right?). But, yes, I want to assure you that everything we discuss in this book *can* be done with twins. This process might take planning, it may take some creativity, but I promise you, if you follow our advice, your twinnies will eventually sleep great.

However, I want to gently let you know that there really are no one-size-fits-all solutions. You may need to try multiple strategies to find the one or ones that work. That's part of why it is important to read not only the chapter on the age your twinnies are today but also the chapters covering the previous two months of age if you can. If one sleep strategy worked across the board for all babies, Kim and I would be millionaires, sitting on a beach with strawberry mojitos in our hands. If there was *one* specific age that was the *best* age to start sleep coaching, the first few pages would say, "Start this many days after your twins are born," and TA-DA, everyone is sleeping. The end!

While you figure out what works for you, Kim and I will be here, holding your hand through each of these pages and making sure that your twinnies are well cared for, that you are well cared for, and that you understand the why behind our recommendations. I don't want you to say, "Nat's gone nuts! How the heck am I going to do XYZ with twins?" I got you! We will get through this together. Trust me. OK?

Reading the First Five Months

One final note: If you are absolutely exhausted and need to immediately address a specific sleep issue, you can pop right to the month and/or subsection that will help you most. But once you've learned a technique that can help, I highly recommend going back and reading the entire book, starting with chapter 2, "Before Delivery Day." We share many baby-related nuggets throughout that help support sleep from all different angles. For example, you may first zero in on a technique in "Your Twins' Third Month" that helps you extend your twins' first stretch of night sleep. But after trying this solution, go back and start the book at the beginning—even though your kids may have passed some of the milestones we highlight. The techniques in earlier chapters can also (almost always) be implemented later and will create the strongest possible foundation for sleep coaching once your twins are developmentally ready.

OK, It's Time to Begin!

Are you ready? Are you already tired? Don't worry, we'll help you get some sleep soon. We genuinely hope that this book gives you and your family everything you need to create a better home for all of you. Let's get started, shall we?

————

Notes

_____

_____

_____

_____

_____

_____

_____

_____

_____

_____

_____

_____

_____

_____

_____

_____

_____

chapter two

Before Delivery Day

Believe it or not, you can start the entire sleep coaching process before your twins get here. Create an ideal sleep area for your kiddos while you're still expecting and put yourself one step ahead on the whole sleep process.

However, a lot in this chapter is about you. Kim and I find that many other pediatric sleep books only talk about the babies. They don't address the most important factor—YOU! And honestly, not just you, but your whole support system. Your entire family will contribute to your twins' sleep coaching adventure. It takes a village, right? Well, let's get that village prepared!

Preparing for Your Twins' Arrival

The final months before your twins arrive is your chance to gather any items you'd like to have at the ready to help you nurture and protect their sleep. New parents often joke that all they *really* need in the first few months are diapers, wipes, and a good stroller, yet some other items become indispensable! Many of our Twiniversity parents rely heavily on a twin bassinet and a double breastfeeding pillow, for example.

Folks often hyperfocus on "stuff" during their nesting phase, and trust me, we are all about it over here! "Stuff" is something you have total control over. So, using this time to get your home ready with all the gear you'll need for your twinnies is fantastic. (Just a word to the wise: Create a budget. We've watched families spend WAY too much on stuff only to have to make trips to UPS or the baby store with returns.)

We have an entire "Multiple Birth Necessities" sheet for you over on our website that takes all the guesswork out of a twin baby registry. We sort it by Must Have, Nice to Have, Borrow, Skip It. You can also check out our latest product recommendations to make twin life easier in our Twiniversity "Twins Gear Guide" or join us for a Twiniversity "Expecting Twins" class. You can access all of these via the QR code.

FAST for You

When we look at FAST in future months, we'll be talking about your twins. This month, we're looking at you!

Food = Fuel for You and Your Twinnies

True, you're not breastfeeding or bottle-feeding your twinnies *yet*, but of course, when you have some buns in the oven, you are already providing your twins much-needed fuel. Eating during a twin pregnancy can pose quite a challenge. Sometimes their tiny feet might be positioned in such a way that it honestly makes it tough to eat. Even if all you can manage is throwing a couple of almonds in your mouth, you really do need to focus on nutrition. Oh, and not just nutrition, but staying hydrated as well. We've had *way* too many Twiniversity families end up in labor and delivery thinking they were having contractions when they were just dehydrated. So, drink your water!

If you are planning on breastfeeding your duo, stay extra vigilant about your nutrition after delivery, too. If you aren't eating, and ideally eating properly, you're not going to feel like your best self, and that's what we'll need from you every day. Raising twins is an around-the-clock job. You can't live on coffee and doughnuts. You'll need some real protein, good carbs, great fiber, and nutritious goodies to get you through the day. (Keep in mind, though, you'll need an extra five hundred calories a day if you are breastfeeding twins! So just say yes to that doughnut!)

Feeding is one of the pillars that supports your twinnies' daily sleep, and the same goes for you. Please don't ignore what you're doing with your diet because you get a bit busy with the twins after they arrive.

Attachment: Bonding Before Birth

Often, when I meet with expectant parents of twins, they are worried that they won't have any "natural instincts." They are stressed they won't know how to respond to their babies or be able to understand them. I'll gently remind you that these babies are new to not only you and your family but also the world. It will take a little time to learn how best to support and connect with them. Over time, as you all get to know each other, your confidence will grow and those instinctual nurturing feelings will show up.

But there are also things you can do ahead of time to increase your bond with them, either while pregnant or, if you're adopting or using a surrogate, while waiting for your babies to be born. For some birth mothers, an attachment forms as soon as you get that positive pregnancy test. But others, as well as partners and adoptive/surrogate parents, bond with their twins in other ways, like by imagining what they will be like when they join the family. As you wait for your duo to arrive, sit in their room and envision the life that is wonderfully waiting in front of you.

Believe it or not, that strong attachment you're creating will support your kiddos' healthy sleep. If your children feel secure, sleep—and honestly, the rest of your parenting journey—will be simpler and more rewarding.

The Past Is Not the Future

When a family is expecting, parents often reflect on their own childhood. Don't be surprised if you find that good and bad memories start popping into your head. With those memories will come emotions. The trick is to acknowledge these emotions while keeping them from interfering with how you care for and nurture your babies.

Not everyone was lucky enough to grow up with a *Brady Bunch* kinda lifestyle, where there was a snack on the table after school and you played football with your pops on the weekend. You should remember, though, that this is *your* opportunity to parent, and you can make *any* changes you'd like.

I often discuss this during our Twiniversity class; I call it a "parenting do-over." It's your chance to create the childhood and life that maybe you wanted yourself. That's the amazing thing about life. Every day that the sun comes up is another opportunity to make things awesome for us and those around us.

If your own childhood was picture perfect, you might want to start thinking about the traditions that made you happy and how to pass those on within your own family. If your childhood was less than ideal, you may want to have a heart-to-heart talk with your partner and tell them about it. If you are worried about history repeating itself in a negative way, this is also your opportunity to reach out and ask for help. It's amazing how much baggage we carry with us throughout our lives. Let's try to unpack some of the heavy stuff before your duo arrives so you'll start this amazing twin adventure with less on your shoulders.

A Note on Trauma

We all know how important it is to take care of your body during a pregnancy, but we often neglect to take care of our minds. If you have had any traumatic events you haven't yet healed from, or if you have, or do, suffer from anxiety or depression, it's doubly important that you take care of yourself during pregnancy and after. Put your twins and their sleep aside here for a moment. Take this time to find the support that you need right now, or perhaps line up a few practitioners you can speak with if/when you need them.

If you don't want to do it for yourself, do it for your twins. Taking care of your own mind will help you be more attuned to your little ones' needs. It will have a direct correlation with good, quality sleep for them and you. And healthy sleep is a form of healing in itself.

Soothing: Taking Care of You

Babies aren't the only ones who benefit from soothing—you do, too! Expecting families often get caught up in stress over doctors' appointments, choosing the right gear, and overall anxiety about the big change in their life, but it's so important that you step outside of all that to take care of the person who matters most today: *you*! Without "you," there is no "them."

Some self-care activities might be second nature to you already. If you're stressed from a tough day at work, you might call a friend for support, go for a walk, or practice some deep breathing to calm yourself. In the first several months of your babies' lives, some of these actions might not be as available to you once you're responsible for those tiny two and not just yourself anymore. Because of that, you'll want to figure out some strategies for self-care that's doable when you're not alone and you need it.

Self-care isn't just for after your little ones are born, and practicing ways to relieve your stress now will pay off dividends in your future. Did you know that right now, during pregnancy, your stress level is impacting your twins? Regular stress in the last trimester can cause birth mothers to release stress chemicals called cortisol and glutamate that can be passed on to their babies. It turns out that particularly stressed birth mothers can also have babies who, once born, cry more. Yeah, let's try to skip the "crying more" portion of your twinnies' early days.

Women tend to be accustomed to being the caregivers, which often means putting others before themselves. But taking time for yourself is an unselfish thing to do. Your well-being is SO, SO important to not only your babies but also everyone around you. Moms expecting twins often experience more stress than a typical singleton mom. Our pregnancies can be a bit higher risk, cause our bodies to work overtime, and be exhausting overall. Emotionally and physically, twin pregnancies can really wreak havoc. Please consider breaking this cycle. Sure, there will be plenty of times that you'll have to focus on the kiddos first, but for now, during your pregnancy, take some time and focus on you—and use this time, too, to think about how you can keep taking care of yourself even after your twins are here.

We reached out to our favorite experts for ideas to help you take care of your mind, body, and spirit when your babies are young, and these appear throughout the book. Here, we just want to remind you how important it will be to make time to soothe yourself, in addition to your babies.

Stop Shoulding on Yourself

I once recorded a Twiniversity podcast episode, number 107 to be exact, with Fran Pitre, a mom of twins times three. Yup. Times THREE! I'll give you a moment to let that sink in. She has three sets of twins: boy/boy, girl/girl, and boy/girl. She's someone I've known for well over a decade and someone I've always looked up to. Her big takeaway in the episode was that we need to stop using the word *should* when it comes to our lives, our children, and our futures. What other people do is not what you "should" do. You have to create the path that is best for you, no matter if it's in parenting, breastfeeding, your delivery day, your pregnancy, or anything else you can think of. Thinking of what should be can lead to epic amounts of unnecessary stress and anxiety. So yeah, skip the shoulding on yourself, OK?

Temperament: Time for Some Self-Reflection

Before you meet your babies, it is helpful to get to know your own temperament. For example, how sensitive are you to crying and noises? Does change bother you? Your understanding of your temperament and your partner's temperament will help you better relate to and understand your babies, as well as your own reactions and feelings toward them.

Take a moment to have a conversation with your partner about how you perceive your own temperament and how they perceive theirs. Please be sensitive. This isn't an attack on anyone's personality but an exercise in self-awareness.

Who's Who?

Learning your twins' unique temperaments is one of your first opportunities to see them as separate individuals. It's often unofficially noticed, even in utero, that Baby A has a stronger will while Baby B is more go with the flow. Once you deliver, it's important to take note of their individual cues—and to do that, you'll need to have a system in place to tell them apart, especially if they are identical twins or even just the same sex. You have to be able to know who is who!

You'll want to come up with a system during your pregnancy that you can implement as soon as they arrive. Some families use nontoxic nail polish on one twin's toes; others dress one twin in a particular color all the time. Some use ankle bracelets with each child's name on them, while others have "assigned seating," meaning that one is always on the left and the other on the right. (Having a fool-proof way of telling them apart isn't just for you and your sanity in those early days before you get to know them. It's for anyone else caring for your children. Parents might be able to know which kiddo is which immediately, but Grandma or Aunt Pam may have a much harder time.)

Preparing for a Good Enough Night's Sleep

As your twin delivery day approaches, we recommend that you focus on getting a good amount of sleep yourself, setting up a sleep-friendly nursery or other sleeping areas, and preparing for sleep disruptions when they arrive—because they *will* arrive.

Counting Your Own Sleep Sheep

Try to get as much sleep as possible during your pregnancy. I know it's tough to get a full eight hours of sleep between getting up to go to the bathroom 17,000 times a night and the babies having a full-on dance party in your belly at 2 AM, but do what you can. Also, studies suggest that pregnancy causes an increase in REM sleep (particularly in the third trimester) and a decrease in deep sleep. This means you'll get more opportunities for some fun dreams about your sweet babies on the way, but potentially less deep sleep, which is the restorative part of sleep, and so feel less refreshed than you'd like. Plus, pregnant women can *feel* sleepier, regardless of the amount of sleep they are getting, because of the amount of progesterone in their bodies—and the fact that their bodies are taking care of three humans at the same time.

Here are some things you can try to get some more rest when you're pregnant with your twinnies:

1. Finish drinking the recommended amount of water (as per your OB) before 7 PM. You'll need fewer overnight trips to the bathroom.

2. Invest in a good maternity pillow. You might even want to consider taking your twins' breastfeeding pillow out of the package before the kids arrive. Many moms find that it provides good back support while resting in bed.

3. Find your spot! If you were a back sleeper and now you are forced to be a side sleeper because of the babies' positions, consider putting props around you so you avoid rolling. Perhaps put a pillow against your back so that, if you try to roll, you can't.

4. If bed isn't working out for you anymore . . . move! Not out of your house but out of your bedroom. Try the couch, a recliner, a dining room chair—nothing is off limits. It's your home and you need to make yourself more comfortable, so try it all out.

5. Get consistent rest. Ideally, I'd love it if you had a regular bedtime. You don't have to literally close your eyes at that time, but you should start winding down from your day. If you typically go to bed at 11 PM, get in bed at 10 or even 9:30. Use that time to relax, meditate, write in your journal, or anything else that puts you in a good headspace for sleep. DO NOT—I repeat DO NOT—get on your phone. The light emitted from your phone can trigger your brain into thinking it's daytime! So put the phone, the tablet, and even the e-reader down. Consider even turning off the TV. Darkness equals good sleep, so make it dark and let your mind relax and unwind.

A healthy sleep schedule for your twins starts now. I know it's hard to believe, but a pregnant mother regulates her baby's sleep in utero—so sticking to a healthy sleep schedule can help your babies. too.

Planning for Overnights

You can also start to think about what your nights might look like once your babies arrive and create a loose plan to support not only your twins but also you and your partner—so that you both are getting enough sleep as well.

Overnight Help

Many families of twins seek additional overnight help when they arrive home from the hospital. Sometimes it's a grandma or sister-in-law who chip in for a bit, or it could even be a paid nanny.

If you are getting overnight help, you need to be sure about your plan for sleeping arrangements. Will you have the babies sleep in your room (see the section on room sharing, page 31) and have your helper come into your room to assist with feeds and diaper changes? Are you comfortable with that? Is your partner? Is your helper? You'll need to discuss that so there is no guessing what your expectations are each night.

It's especially important to create a plan you are comfortable with if you plan on breastfeeding. Breastfeeding twins is an around-the-clock job, and you will need to get up every two to three hours to feed them or pump. Your helper has to be on board with that and willing to either (1) wake you up so that you can go to where the babies are, or (2) bring the babies to you regularly throughout the night—meaning they will have to come into your room where you and your partner may be sound asleep. Also, if your partner is a light sleeper and you're going to be breastfeeding next to them, this may be an issue. Look at your overnight plan from all angles before you make any concrete decisions.

It's been my experience that if you hire an overnight "baby nurse" (who odds are is not, and has never been, an RN, something some parents are surprised by), they tend to be a bit stricter about staying on schedule and may not be as willing to bring you the babies to feed in the middle of the night, since it's simpler to just bottle-feed. Be extra cautious when hiring any outside assistance and be sure to set clear boundaries and expectations when it comes to caring for your twins overnight (or any other time of day).

If you are lucky enough to have a friend or family member who can assist you even one night a week, snatch that up! Caring for twins is challenging enough during the day; nighttime presents its own issues, especially when you're sleep deprived. Even with family or friends, lay out a clear plan of how you'd like the night to go; they will not want to upset or disappoint you.

Help Me!

If you feel that you just can't manage this alone anymore, don't worry; help is not far away. Many types of help are available, from traditional nannies to au pairs, and we want to ensure that you know all your options before you choose. Twiniversity has compiled a great resource page for just this topic, which you can access using the QR code. Heck, we'll even give you a PDF filled with nanny interview questions. And if you are heading back to work and putting your twinnies in daycare, we'll cover that as well.

Overnight Feedings

When it comes to feeding your twinnies overnight, there are a few options to consider, depending on whether you're planning to breastfeed or bottle-feed. For the sake of simplicity, I'm going to create three roles here: the mom, the partner, and the assistant.

Option A: Your partner or assistant changes one baby, then brings them to you for a feeding at your breast while your partner or assistant changes and bottle-feeds (with either previously pumped breast milk or formula) the other baby. Your partner or assistant retrieves the baby from you after the feeding and you go back to sleep.

Option B: Your partner or assistant comes into the room with both babies after changing them, and you put them both to breast for a feeding. Your partner can burp one, when it's time, while you burp the other. After you finish the tandem feeding, your partner takes them back to bed.

Option C: Your partner or assistant wakes you up to pump twenty minutes before it's time to feed the babies. You pump and give them your expressed milk. They then use the expressed breast milk to feed one or both babies (depending on your production) and you go back to sleep.

Option D: Your partner or assistant bottle-feed both babies with either previously pumped breast milk from the fridge or formula, while you sleep.

It's encouraged that you take into account your personal sleep habits when you start making your overnight plans. One parent might be a night owl while another might love waking at the crack of dawn. That would make a best-case scenario: Each of you can be "on the clock" during your favorite times of the day.

Perinatal Mood and Anxiety Disorders (PMAD)

We have to talk. Please, we need your full attention—and then when you're done reading this, hand it to your partner for them to read as well.

Many folks have heard of the "baby blues," which may occur the first few weeks after delivery and are typically categorized as brief episodes of mild mood changes. These are extremely common, experienced by 50 to 80 percent of new moms. But the baby blues are transient. They go away in about two weeks. If they don't, you may be dealing with something more serious: Perinatal Mood and Anxiety Disorders (PMAD).

Under the PMAD umbrella there are six specific disorders: postpartum bipolar disorder, postpartum panic disorder, postpartum obsessive-compulsive disorder, postpartum psychosis, postpartum post-traumatic stress disorder, and the most familiar, postpartum depression.

A PMAD affects up to one in seven new moms, according to the Children's Center of Philadelphia. Read more about PMAD, and how to recognize it, on page 103.

If sad feelings or anxiety are overwhelming, if you experience any thoughts of harming yourself or your baby, or if your symptoms start to interfere with your daily life, get evaluated for postpartum depression and other postpartum disorders immediately. If necessary, call 911.

It's also important for the people close to new parents to be on the lookout for symptoms of a PMAD. Parents experiencing postpartum depression don't always recognize the signs or may already be too depressed to take action.

PMADs are completely treatable when the right help is provided. If you or your partner is experiencing signs of a PMAD, please contact your doctor and check out Postpartum Support International (postpartum.net).

Creating a Safe Sleep-Friendly Environment for Your Twins

One of the most exciting things new parents do is set up their duo's nursery. While you're having all that fun, it's important to make sure that you are not just creating a beautiful social media–ready aesthetic, if that's your goal, but also making your twins' space as safe and sleep friendly as possible.

First, make sure that the area is safe. A safe sleep environment includes a safe sleeping area and a safe room. Your twins' nursery should have:

- A crib with a correctly sized mattress, with no gaps on any side, and snuggly fitted sheets.
- Nothing else in the crib. No pillows. No blankets. No toys.
- An appropriate temperature of between 68 and 72 degrees.
- No loose wires around the crib.
- No hanging cords within arm's reach of your twins.
- Securely fastened decorative items.
- Correctly secured dressers, changing tables, shelves, and any other items that can be fastened to a wall.
- Baby-safe covers on all outlets.
- No tripping hazards, like throw rugs.
- A correctly working smoke detector and carbon monoxide detector.
- No within-reach baby creams and lotions; they should be safely secured.

These are just SOME of the items you need to watch out for when creating a safe sleep area for your newborn twins. If you are stressed that your nursery may not be safe enough, feel free to check out our Twiniversity "Complete Baby Safety" course or call a local babyproofer in your area. You might also consider checking with the social worker at your local hospital for additional resources. They are a good go-to source for most things baby related and will be more than happy to help you.

A healthy sleep environment is not only safe but also calm and comforting and not overstimulating and noisy. Younger babies can often sleep anywhere during the day (though not all of them, of course!), but they might sleep best in their individual sleep space at night. The sleep environment that your twins need will be based on their individual temperaments, so you may have to experiment a bit to find the environment that works best.

Our suggestions for a more sleep-friendly space:

- A soothing room color, decorations, and fixtures.
- Room-darkening shades to control the amount of light in the room.
- A dim night-light. When you're feeding and caring for your babies in the middle of the night, you'll want enough light to see what you're doing—particularly if you're changing a diaper—but not so much light that it completely "wakes" the kids (or you!). A yellow or orange (a.k.a. low blue) light is ideal. You can experiment with turning the dim night-light off while your babies sleep and keeping it on to determine which works best for everyone involved.
- A white noise machine. We recommend trying white noise with all babies, but it is a must for babies who need a little extra sleep support, as it can help to block out noises throughout the rest of the house and outside their room window. You'll learn more about white noise in "Your Twins' First Month" on page 76. An alternative to white noise is quiet, calming music or lullabies, which can work better for some babies, especially at bedtime. Be ready to experiment once your twinnies arrive.

For specific current sleep gear recommendations, refer to our "Twins Gear Guide" using the QR code.

Room Sharing with Your Twins

Room sharing is when your newborns sleep on an independent sleep surface like a twins' co-sleeper, twin bassinet, or twin pack and play in their parents' room for easy access and safety. (This is not the same thing as co-cribbing, which is discussed on page 34.) Some families plan to room share just for the first few weeks, while they are learning the ropes, while others plan for six months or longer. The time limit is up to you and what you're most comfortable with.

Having your duo sleep safely next to you—literally at your fingertips—so that you can reach over and touch them might give you peace of mind. For moms who have had C-sections and have difficulty getting up and moving around for the first few weeks, this setup can be particularly helpful if there aren't extra pairs of hands around to get the babies when you want or need them. However, you'll want to be sure that any sleeping vessel that you have set up for the twins fits in your room without blocking doorways or windows in case of an emergency. Parents of singletons typically need to worry less about this because a singleton bassinet or co-sleeper is usually much smaller than what our kiddos need to safely sleep. So, consider your surroundings.

Also, make sure that you have a backup plan or two in case room sharing doesn't work out. Sometimes it's not because of lack of space but because it doesn't really work well for either you or your babies. You might find that one of your twins is particularly sensitive to your partner's snoring, or you are unable to sleep because you pop up every time you hear one of them stir. Your backup plan may be moving the bassinet into another room and even having one parent sleep on a separate mattress next to them. Make sure you have discussed your room sharing plans with your partner and are making choices that support your whole family's well-being. If you or your partner want some space from the babies, hear each other out, and decide what you can do to make sure everyone is on the same page and can get the best possible night's sleep.

If you do plan to share a room with your twinnies, whether for the first few weeks or longer, you'll want to set your space up so that you don't make a lot of noise when you go to bed. Be sure there isn't anything to trip over and that you don't have to squeeze through small spaces. The small space squeezing is especially an issue if you have a C-section! Let's remember that your incision will be healing and you'll need to be extra, extra, extra careful.

Co-Sleeping

OK, we have to talk about this. There are so many controversies within the parenting world and if I had to rank them, I'd say that co-sleeping would be in the top three. I'm not saying you should or shouldn't co-sleep. I'm saying you need to do what's best for your family. And while I'd love if this book could answer this big ol' question for you, co-sleeping is a heavily debated topic in the United States.

If you're planning to co-sleep with your twinnies, you need to be absolutely sure that your sleep space is ready for your babies. Please do your due diligence and speak to those who care for you and/or for your babies about co-sleeping in general and how to do it safely with two if that's your choice.

Some parents end up co-sleeping out of sheer desperation; we call these reactive co-sleepers. The first few months of your twins' lives can be a time of utter sleep deprivation for everyone, and parents can end up co-sleeping because they are understandably doing the best they can to get their kids and themselves as much sleep as possible. Usually, the twins have their own sleep space, but the parents bring the babies (or maybe even just one baby) into their bed during particularly fussy periods throughout the night.

If you notice that you are doing things you wouldn't typically do to cope with your sleep deprivation, and you feel like it's too much of a struggle, you NEED to ask for help.

This isn't a "want," this is a need.

Having a baby is a big challenge, and twins . . . it's much, much, much more challenging, and it's easy to make mistakes. Especially overnight, when your body is screaming for you to get some rest. It may not just be overnights, either. If you are exhausted while feeding or nursing on a sofa, you can end up accidentally falling asleep with your baby there, too.

For the record, I'm not trying to make you panic. I'm just trying to make you realize that sleep deprivation is *no* joke! We've heard some pretty sad stories about things that have happened because of parental exhaustion. And we want to help you have as many great, happy stories and as few sad stories as possible.

If you are ever so sleep deprived that you literally cannot keep your eyes open (and don't have another pair of hands to help you), it's OK to put the twins in their safe sleep environment and close your eyes for a moment. You are better off being purposeful about making sure they are safe than accidentally rolling on a baby or having a baby fall. It is OK to ask for help! Say it with me . . . for real. "*It is OK to ask for help."* Louder this time for the people in the back: "IT IS OK TO ASK FOR HELP!"

You cannot be expected to be on call twenty-four hours a day, seven days a week, without a nap or some uninterrupted sleep. Sleep deprivation is REAL and is used as a *literal* form of torture. So yeah, please, make sure you ask for help if you are getting to a dangerous point with your lack of sleep.

One Crib or Two?

While I'd love to just gloss over this topic and whistle nonchalantly as I have you flip to the next page, I know that co-cribbing (your twins sleeping in the same crib) is a HUGE discussion within the multiple-birth community. I have a personal and a professional stance on this, and I'd like you to hear me out on both.

Neither Kim nor I will ever advise you on what "should" be done here, but we do want to present the options and the research so that you can make an educated call on what to do in your own home with your own twins. Our word is not law, and at this time, neither is anyone else's. Also, at no time do we expect you to follow our advice if it interferes with what your pediatrician advises you, ever! If you're interested in crib sharing, please discuss it at length with your health care practitioner and get their opinion on what is best for your twins; they are the ones who know their whole life story.

When I first wrote *What to Do When You're Having Two*, I had a lengthy conversation with my editor on what we should do about this entire co-cribbing discussion. In the United States and many other countries around the globe, twin co-cribbing was standard practice up until the 1990s, when the American Academy of Pediatrics (AAP) released new sleep guidelines for twins. Since then, practitioners around the country have been specifically recommending that twins DO NOT crib share—that they should sleep separately at all times.

Being that I'm the big cheese of the largest group of twins families in the world, I felt it was my duty to dig into this research myself back in 2018. I was very confused to find that while the AAP made this recommendation to hundreds of thousands of families, their research about twin sleeping arrangements was not specifically done using research about twins. If you are sitting there scratching your head: yup. Join the club.

So, back then, I reached out to the AAP public relations team and received this back:

> As I understand it, there is not a whole lot of data about co-bedding of multiples. The technical report contains all of the references that AAP uses. The recommendation came from the references and then from the bed-sharing data that show that sibling bed sharing is dangerous.

I reached out again recently and received a note back that their recommendations for twins remain the same—despite the fact that it's not fair, or often practical, to tell twin families to abide by rules made for siblings rather than twins specifically. Siblings could mean a ten-year-old and a six-month-old. Yes, that they shouldn't sleep in the same bed makes perfect sense. But twins?

Honestly, I dug into this so deeply because my own twins were co-cribbed in the NICU by their doctors and nurses during their stay there. I found that my children, at least, slept much better when they were near each other. In fact, while we were in the NICU (fourteen days for Baby B and thirty-one days for Baby A), I also witnessed, several times, how their heartbeats and respiration would often sync up when they were next to each other (yes, it was a bit creepy!). I personally felt that my own twins were stronger together than apart. But that's just me.

I know I'm kinda leaving you hanging here. I can't say, "Your twins *should* sleep in the same crib" because then I'm going against what our biggest regulating body of pediatric doctors recommends. I also can't say, "Your twins should *never* sleep in the same crib" because so many families feel it's better for their children, and this practice is still common throughout many parts of the world.

I recommend checking the latest recommendations for twins for yourself on the American Academy of Pediatrics website, AAP.org, and then speaking to your twins' health care practitioner to see what they personally recommend for your twins' sleeping arrangements.

FAST to Sleep Summary

What to Focus on Before Your Babies Arrive

1. Take care of yourself:
   - Make sure you are filling your belly with good nutritious treats, but splurge as often as your doc allows. You deserve to be spoiled as much as possible!
   - Consider how your past might affect your future.
   - Stop shoulding on yourself.
   - Reflect your own temperament and how it might play a role in your upcoming life as a new parent.
   - Evaluate your self-care routine.
2. Prepare for better sleep:
   - Decide with your partner where your children will sleep.
   - Create a safe and sleep-friendly environment for your twins.
   - Create a plan for overnights.

Notes

_____

_____

_____

_____

_____

_____

_____

_____

_____

_____

_____

_____

chapter three

Your Twins' First Month

Ages Birth to 4 Weeks

This month, you'll learn about how your babies are operating from their primitive brain and about how you, as a parent, are experiencing changes that let you better care for your twins. (Remember to take adjusted age into consideration, especially when it comes to sleep.)

Happy birth day! Yes, this month will be a little chaotic, but that's not always a bad thing. For the first time, you'll get to look at your twins, with all those tiny fingers and toes, and be in absolute awe of Mother Nature.

Starting with a NICU Vacation?

My twins got here a bit on the early side. Born at thirty-four weeks on the day, they didn't feel like my husband, John, should have his own birthday anymore, so they arrived a little after 5 AM on his birthday. Yup. Best! Gift! Giver! Ever! (Or worst. Depends on how you look at it.)

My Baby A's first month was spent in the NICU, while my Baby B was there for a quick fourteen days. A NICU stay is something that's more common than folks think! Up to 80 percent of twin families spend at least a couple of hours there with one or both of their kiddos after their birth. There are a lot of things that may not have finished "cooking" if you delivered early, and the NICU is where a hospital can closely mimic that in utero experience with tools like oxygen and feeding tubes.

As a NICU graduate mom, I can tell you that the thirty-one days we spent there after my twins' delivery day left me with mixed emotions. Initially, I almost dreaded going into the NICU because, to me, it was a reminder that my body couldn't handle the stress of my twin pregnancy and that my babies couldn't be right there beside me. All that wasted sadness and guilt. I wish that I'd known then what I know now: that I couldn't have prevented my preterm labor. I also wish I'd known how much I would eventually learn to love the NICU. I had no idea I would get unlimited support from the amazing nurses and staff. In hindsight, the NICU was one of the most extraordinary experiences of my life. I had some of the best experts in the world at my fingertips to answer questions, show me techniques, and offer me encouragement.

The NICU is covered at length in my first book, *What to Do When You're Having Two*, in our Twiniversity classes, and on our website, but I'll sum up a few important tidbits here for making the NICU experience a lot easier, whether you're spending your first days, weeks, or even months there.

1. Use the staff pediatricians, neonatologists, and specialists in your hospital while your babies are still admitted to the NICU. If you call your pediatrician from home, they will be visiting your twinnies only before or after office hours, making it harder for you to communicate with them if you have questions while you're visiting.

2. You can ask to have a primary nurse—one nurse who is specifically assigned to your baby or babies. Having a primary nurse means you'll have one point person to deal with each day.

3. Find out what services are offered by your delivery hospital's social workers. You might be eligible to stay at a local Ronald McDonald house once you are discharged to be closer to your babies, you might

be able to take a hospital CPR class before your twins are discharged, and more. Some states even have grants available for families who have children in the NICU to assist with mortgage and car payments, so that all family members can care for their new tiny tots.

4. Your friends and family might feel a little lost because they don't know how to help you. Ask them to send meals and snacks and take care of your pets if you have them—these are some of the most extraordinary things they can do for you at this time. The babies will have an immense amount of support, so your family should spend the time focusing on you and your partner, and your emotional well-being.

5. Ask for help, please. Here in the United States, many NICUs don't always ask moms the right questions to check for any postpartum mood disorders, something that's typically done in a pediatric office during your first postdelivery visit. Since your twins' first doctor's appointment might be with the staff at the hospital, any mood issues you're having might get overlooked. Please promise me that you'll try your hardest to remain open and communicative with your partner, your best friend, or whoever else you find to be a good listener. If you are anxious, sad, upset, and/or confused, don't "take one for the team." Reach out to anyone, no matter if you think they can help or not. Just keep talking. If you don't speak up, no one will know what you are going through, and therefore they can't help. If you have no one that you think will listen, you have an entire community to support you at Twiniversity, now and always.

You can access Twiniversity's NICU resources at the QR code.

Home at Last

Get your camera ready! Homecoming day for your twin or twins will be one you'll most likely never forget. Many moms remember what time of the day they were discharged from the hospital, what they wore, and how the family got home. It's all so exciting.

With all that excitement, you might be a teeny-tiny bit overwhelmed. OK, let's be honest, you'll probably feel more than a tiny bit overwhelmed. It's a lot. Trust me, I know. I feel ya. It's like twins magically appeared in your living room and are now expecting YOU to take care of them. Even with all the preparation in the world, it still feels shocking.

I'm going to take a wild guess here and say that you're also feeling pretty wiped out. Delivering twins is no joke, my friend! And now that they are here, sleep may be the last thing on your mind because of all the other things you have to do in a day—not to mention you might be breastfeeding them around the clock. Your endorphins have probably kicked in, and you may feel like you're running on auto-pilot during those early weeks. It may be a blur to you later, but while you are in the eye of that storm, it can be stressful, to say the least.

For this first month, we're going to cover newborn sleep, but we also want you to learn what your newborns are going through (both mentally and physically) to have realistic expectations for what they are capable of. Understanding what is going on at this stage helps you know that you are not failing as a parent when your babies are not sleeping ten hours at a time or achieving other milestones expected at their age.

 ## Your Developing Duo

Your babies' developmental milestones fall into four main categories: *motor*, *sensory*, *communication*, and *feeding*. This month, we'll look at your babies' brain development and their automatic reflexes, among others.

Knowing when your babies will reach particular milestones will help you understand their behaviors, as well as how to soothe them. It also lets you know when to implement various aspects of sleep shaping. As I shared in chapter 1, this gentle practice uses nighttime and daytime habits to lay a foundation for better sleep, so when your twinnies are ready, they can more easily learn how to put themselves to sleep and stay asleep. This is something your babies will slowly learn how to do over the next several months. It's not an instant process. So please be patient with them and with yourself.

The Fourth Trimester

The fourth trimester, or the first three months after the birth of your twinnies, is a time of incredible growth and ideally a period when we can mimic a womb-like environment to help our babies continue to grow, develop, and become the best tiny humans they can be. Let's take a closer look at where your sweet tiny baby humans are during this period and why they need your support.

A Note About Adjusted Age Versus Gestational Age

Because your twinnies might have been born earlier than expected, your fourth trimester might be even longer. The majority of our kiddos arrive before that forty-week mark. In fact, over 82 percent of twins born in the US are considered premature (under 37 weeks), according to the CDC's most current research.

If you had your babies prematurely, you'll hear docs asking about what's called "adjusted age." This is the term used to describe how old your babies would be *if* they had been born at term. To calculate your twins' adjusted age, take their due date and subtract the number of weeks they were born early.

I find the more premature your babies are, the longer you'll need to remind your doctors about their adjusted age. Since my twins were born six weeks early, I had to calculate their adjusted age for quite some time. Years, in fact. But looking at milestones based on your babies' adjusted age versus their gestational age (the actual time since they were born) will relieve a lot of stress. My twins were not meeting the milestones of their gestational age but were typically always hitting their adjusted age dates.

Take each day as it comes and speak to your doc often about realistic expectations regarding your particular twinnies.

Brain Development

It may surprise you to learn that most of the human brain develops after birth, not before. During the first year of life, their brains triple in size. Ninety percent of all human brain growth occurs *within the first five years of life.*

Babies (and all humans, for that matter) have three brain regions: the *downstairs (or primitive) brain*, the *emotional brain*, and the *upstairs brain (or neocortex)*, terms coined by neuropsychiatrist and author Dr. Daniel J. Siegel. At this stage, a baby's downstairs brain—which oversees instinctive behavior related to survival and controls essential bodily functions—is all that is "online." Their neocortex—in adults, this is where thinking, remembering, reasoning, and learning happen—is very unfinished. In other words, your newborns are currently completely incapable of these skills.

During the first few months of your twins' lives, they aren't able to reason or figure out how to calm themselves down—and that's where you come in. Your job as a parent is to learn and respond to your kiddos' instinctive behaviors and react accordingly. Your twins are looking for you to respond to their needs.

For example, one twin or the other might be:

- Hungry and need food.
- Sitting in a wet or dirty diaper and need you to change them into a clean one.
- Upset (perhaps because they are uncomfortable) and need your help to calm down.
- Tired and need help falling asleep.
- Overwhelmed by their surroundings and need you to bring them to a quiet room for some chill time.

Although the first two are obviously critical, they're also fairly straightforward. The rest require a bit more explanation and a few definitions.

As you learned in chapter 1, when you're in a calm state, you are considered *regulated*. *Self-regulation* is the ability to monitor and keep your emotions in check. This is not a skill we are born with but rather one we learn, typically around three and a half or four years old, by watching our parents and caregivers.

On the flip side, *dysregulation* occurs when you are unable to manage your emotions and, particularly, your emotional responses. When we find ourselves dysregulated as adults, most of us can quickly bring ourselves back into a regulated state (often subconsciously—we might sigh when frustrated, for example, which is the body's way of taking a deep breath to calm ourselves down).

When your newborn gets dysregulated, your job is to help them get regulated because they are unable to do it on their own yet. Your response helps them calm down in the moment, but it also helps them long term by creating a secure attachment where your children feel safe because they can trust you to respond to them when they need you. This emotionally responsive parenting helps your twins develop the crucial brain connections that assist them in learning to successfully regulate themselves later in life.

We have another job when it comes to regulation and our babies, and that's to help them learn the difference between what it feels like to be regulated and what it feels like to be dysregulated. Allowing them to become overly dysregulated by not responding to their needs can prevent them from learning and recognizing this difference. A baby (or any human, for that matter) in a dysregulated state cannot learn effectively. And this is a time when your twins are learning an incredible number of new skills daily.

I joke a lot with my Twiniversity students about how they have to cut their babies a little slack. I usually remind them that at one month old, they don't know what the sun is, what that thing is making that barking noise, what poop smells like, and about a zillion other things. They are like little aliens arriving on our planet, and it's our job to show them the world. Another big part of our job is to help them feel safe and secure so they can be open to learning all the wonders this world has to offer.

Note that a particularly dysregulated baby can be very difficult to soothe back to a regulated state, which is why reading your baby's cues is important. The sooner you can come in with a soothing response, the easier they will be to soothe. You'll see this a lot in regard to breastfeeding. I often witness moms trying to get a baby to latch when they are in the throes of a total freak-out. Yeah, that's not going to work until everyone is calm, and I do mean everyone. When babies start freaking out, often parents do, too. That's not the way to set a great example. Even if you are freaking out in your head, try to let your body say differently. Take a deep breath yourself and try to get yourself regulated before trying to regulate your babies.

Regaining Birth Weight

Babies can lose as much as 10 percent of their birth weight in the first few days after birth, but if their growth is on track, they will regain the weight and return to their birth weight within two weeks. Some studies show that it's not even fair to take a baby's weight until they are twenty-four hours old because many lose fluids simply because they were overhydrated because of IV fluids given to mom on delivery day. So, try not to stress too much about your babies' birth weights and go with your gut for feeds while in the hospital. If you are especially worried, speak to the nurses or in-hospital lactation consultant.

Newborn Reflexes

Most of your babies' actions in the early months are reflexive, that is, involuntary. These amazing reflexes evolved to keep your babies safe while their brains are still developing. Some of these reflexes will remain for a few months, and others will go away in weeks. And it can be helpful to understand what to expect regarding a few key reflexes related to feeding and soothing in particular.

Sucking Reflex

Appears: Around 36 weeks gestation

Disappears: At 3 months

The sucking reflex is a survival reflex that appears even before birth. After birth, a baby automatically begins to suck when something touches the roof of their mouth. A premature baby (one born before 36 weeks) may have a harder time latching onto a breast or bottle because this reflex hasn't yet fully developed. Newborns also may have a harder time coordinating their sucking reflex when tired. It may be necessary to wake your twinnies in order to feed them so they can suck properly.

Rooting Reflex

Appears: At birth

Disappears: Around 4 months

The rooting reflex helps your babies find their food. If you touch or stroke the corner of a newborn's mouth, you'll see them turn their head toward where that touch came from and open their mouth. Often, lactation professionals and/or nurses will direct a new parent to do this with their nipple or the tip of a bottle's. This instinctive reflex helps a baby get a great latch and hopefully a great meal. Rooting, along with sucking and bringing their hands to their mouth, is a key feeding cue in the first weeks after birth.

Moro Reflex

Appears: At birth

Disappears: At 2 months

Also called the startle reflex, this reflex often occurs when a baby is startled by a loud noise (their own cry can be the loud noise, by the way) or sudden movement. This reflex makes your babies throw back their head and extend their arms and legs, then rapidly bring them back in. This can be accompanied by a loud cry. Swaddling can be very helpful to keep the Moro reflex from waking a startled newborn by keeping their arms close to their body.

Crying

Between weeks three and twelve, most babies go through a particularly fussy period due to a spurt in brain and physical development. During this time, you may find that your newborns cry more than they used to, particularly toward the end of the day. This late-afternoon or early evening fussiness is common for many babies as the stimulation that builds throughout the day becomes too much for them to process and handle. Many call it the witching hour, and it typically starts around 3 or 4 PM. It can be a real doozy with two crying kiddos, so if you have an extra pair of hands handy, this would be a great time to make sure they're available.

Can this witching hour be avoided, one might ask? Well, maybe. If we can keep your twins from getting overstimulated during the day, the witching hour may never even occur. In general, if we can avoid them getting overstimulated, they'll also be easier to put to sleep both for naps and in the evening. Stay tuned for the "Soothing" section, where you'll learn techniques to help.

Habituation

At this stage, your newborns have the ability to screen out sounds and overstimulating situations by going into a protective state called *habituation*, something first written about by Dr. William A. H. Sammons in his book *The Self Calmed Baby* in 1989. He explains how habituation is one of your babies' early coping skills and allows them to, as he put it, "play possum." If/when your babies get overstimulated, they go into a state of habituation and can tune out the world around them. When your babies are habituating, they *appear* to be sleeping deeply, sometimes even pulling their arms and legs in and closing their eyes.

Babies that are habituating spending a great amount of energy tuning out stimulation. While habituation isn't as stressful for babies as remaining awake, it *is* draining. You can usually tell one or both of your twinnies were habituating if they "wake up" fussy, inconsolable, and exhausted after seeming to be asleep in an environment that is noisy or stressful.

Habituation might occur when your babies sleep through being handled by many relatives at a family function, seeming to be passed around easily. Or when they spend the day sleeping in a stroller when you're at a loud playground with your older kids. You'll learn more about how to recognize and soothe your baby before they habituate in the sleep section.

Supporting Development for Better Sleep

For the first month of twins' lives, parents or other caregivers have to do all of the soothing for them. Later, once twins have the skills to soothe themselves even a little bit, they will be better able to calm themselves enough to fall asleep and eventually put themselves back to sleep when they wake in the middle of the night. In the meantime, your job is to support those tiny little beans and help them as they start to develop these skills.

One of the first stops on the self-soothing train (*choo choo*) is the ability to roll over, which allows babies to get into a more comfortable position. Eventually, they will also be able to intentionally move their hand to their mouth and may choose to self-soothe in this way as well. This ability doesn't occur overnight, but rather comes through the development of their core strength. And that means tummy time!

Just remember, tummy time is for daytime. Your babies should always be "back to sleep," meaning they should always sleep on their back.

Tummy Time

Tummy time is discussed a ton at Twiniversity, especially since twins are often born on the earlier side. Reflux is very common with preterm babies, since the esophagus may not have fully finished developing in utero and is not working 100 percent perfectly yet. Sometimes, parents neglect tummy time, worrying that if they do place their kiddos belly down, they will lose their entire feeding. When you do have a tummy time session and notice that happening, please speak to your twinnies' care team and see if they can offer any specific tips for your particular duo and if they feel the benefit of tummy time is a good idea at this stage.

Often folks just gloss right over tummy time, not realizing how important it is for muscle tone, coordination, and growth in general. It's not just playtime; it's important for physical and neurological development, too. Putting your babies on the floor, on their stomach, strengthens their core muscles through movement and attempting to lift and shift their heads around. It actually works nicely with that bonus baby you have because one twin will often try to find their twin as they are flat on their belly. It's very sweet! Especially as they get older, you'll be able to see how they very much know each other and are looking for their other half during these sessions.

Tummy time is important for sleep development simply because the muscle tone (which varies among babies at birth; some babies are born powerlifters, others aren't) and control your little ones gain through tummy time will eventually help them change positions while sleeping, making them less likely to get uncomfortable, wake, and cry out for help.

During the first month, it's recommended that newborns get ***one to five minutes of tummy time, two to three times per day***. A baby doesn't always like to be on their tummy because their head is so heavy at this age, but I suggest that you commit to this small amount of time if you can.

Tummy time is also where *we* first practice helping our babies learn something that might frustrate them a little bit. We practice letting them feel a bit of discomfort as they remain in a position that strengthens their muscles. This supported-learning dance will occur again when you start sleep shaping and sleep coaching your children. Practicing it now will get you all familiar with the process: You will get more comfortable with allowing your twins to feel healthy discomfort, and your kids will trust that they can handle small doses of discomfort while knowing that you are there to support them through it.

ALTERNATE TUMMY TIME POSITIONS

At this age, you can try a few alternatives to traditional tummy time if you are having a lot of trouble.

My favorite alternate tummy time position is what I call sneaky tummy time, and I recommend you do this as often as you can when you remember. It's simple. Lying on a bed, a recliner, or even an office chair that can safely tilt back, put one of your babies on your chest and lean back. You'll see that your baby will try to lift their head up to look around, activating their core and back muscles. Just be careful they don't knock into you; their tiny heads are harder than you think.

You might even want to do this by a window and talk to whoever the lucky twin on your chest is about what you see outside. Encourage your partner to do the same with your other twinnie. It's a fun way to engage with just one of them. Plus, you can double dip, so to speak. If you unbutton your shirt and take off your baby's onesie, you can have some skin-to-skin contact in addition to tummy time.

You can also sit upright and place one of your twins on the flat of your lap. Be sure to hold on to them so they don't squirm off and fall or hurt themself. This flat position might be less frustrating for them than being on the floor because you are so much closer to them.

Make it a fun game with your partner and see who can keep the twin they are responsible for on their tummy the longest. My money's on you!

Access Twiniversity's tummy time guide at the QR code.

 ## Feeding

We're going to focus A LOT on feeding in this chapter because it is the area of your babies' lives that most affects sleep in the first month. Making sure that their feeding is on track goes a *long* way toward helping your little ones sleep. This section shares what "on track" means when it comes to breast milk and formula intake and how to help your little ones (and yourself) if you encounter challenges. And when we say *feeding*, we're talking about breastfeeding, formula feeding with a bottle, and bottle-feeding breast milk—any way that you are keeping your baby well nourished! In our opinion, there is no "right" way to feed a baby, so whatever you choose, Kim and I back you up 100 percent.

Feeding at This Age

The World Health Organization (WHO) suggests that parents practice exclusive breastfeeding from birth through six months. I understand, however, that breastfeeding may simply not be an option for you since breastfeeding twins can be as overwhelming as it gets. You have to do what works best for you and your children. Your pediatrician is a great resource.

If breastfeeding is a priority for you, you should also consider hiring a twin-specific lactation consultant. They're harder to find, but we have resources for you at Twiniversity, no worries. If you don't have access to a twin-specific lactation person, any Certified Lactation Consultant (CLC) or International Board Certified Lactation Consultant (IBLC) might still do the trick. Just make sure you are very expressive about what your breastfeeding goals are and how willing you are to get there.

That said, my own babies had PLENTY of formula because of my breastfeeding challenges. There is no shame in my game, so I'm always the first to say, "Wanna breastfeed? Cool. Don't want to breastfeed? Cool. Want to breastfeed a little? Cool." For real—as the saying goes, fed is best.

How Much Milk Should My Babies Have?

It's helpful to remember that all babies are different—some like to snack often, while others drink more at a time and go longer between feedings. However, most babies will drink more and go longer between feedings as they grow bigger and their tummies can hold more milk.

Think of your babies' bellies like their gas tanks. You couldn't go on a cross-country road trip if your gas tank only held a cup of gas. Your babies' bellies will grow with time (and along with your milk supply if you are breastfeeding). In the meantime, they have super tiny gas tanks, and that is why they need to eat so often. They need to keep filling up to grow, play, and yes, sleep. Would you be able to sleep if you were hungry? Odds are, no.

In the first month it's recommended that newborns eat ***every two to three hours*** or ***eight to twelve times every twenty-four hours***. Yes, both babies—and that could be twenty-four feeds a day. Welcome to our world.

Each baby might only take in half an ounce per feeding for the first day or two of life, but after that, they will usually drink one to two ounces at each feeding. This amount usually increases to two to three ounces by two weeks of age, but that really depends on your babies. Your pediatrician can guide you in the right direction when it comes to feeding amounts. You have to find that sweet spot: You want to make sure you fill their tiny gas tanks, but you don't want to overfill them because then they could end up spitting up.

The amount your babies need is also weight dependent. How much gas does it take to get their particular car across the finish line? And yes, this means that your twins might be eating two different amounts. It happens. This is one of the important reasons you need to look at your twins as individuals with the same birthday rather than as "the same."

We have a chart on Twiniversity regarding how much milk your babies should be getting, which you can get to using the QR code. But basically, it's a fairly simple calculation:

Body weight (in pounds) × 2.5 = number of ounces they should eat per day

To find the average amount your baby should be eating per feed, you then need to take that number and divide it by the number of feeds they typically have in a day.

Clearly this isn't as doable when exclusively feeding at the breast, but it's pretty simple for bottles. For example, if you have a six-pound baby eating eight times a day . . .

6 × 2.5 = 15 ounces of milk per day
15/8 = about 2 ounces of milk per feeding

Feeding is going well if:

- Your twins are eating (breast or bottle) eight or more times within a twenty-four-hour period (remember: *eight or more in twenty-four*).
- Your breasts feel empty after their feeding (if breastfeeding).
- Your twins have soiled diapers throughout the day. Ideally, it's great if they have three or four poops a day by day four and every day thereafter. It's good to keep track of their poops and pees so you know who did what and when.
- They are relaxed and content after feeding.
- Your babies have strong cries, meaning they have energy and are well fed. Yup, that's a good sign!

If Your Babies Seem Hungrier Than Usual

When your babies are born, their stomachs are each the size of a cherry. At one week old, a baby's stomach has grown to the size of an egg, which means that they can eat more in a feeding. Remember that gas tank analogy? Since their gas tanks are getting bigger, they can hold more gas and go further on that road trip.

If you notice that your babies are hungrier than usual, it's OK to raise the amount you are feeding them or give them a few more minutes at the breast. Most babies experience some type of growth spurt within the first few weeks of life. (This reminds me to remind you: Take tons of pictures. They will grow like little weeds over the first few months.)

Supporting Sleep Through Feeding

Your twinnies need to have a full belly so they can feel content and get some rest. Meeting their feeding needs is one of the most important things you can do to help them get the sleep they need at this age. It's time we jump into the bits and pieces of sleep and how it goes hand in hand with feeding. Ready to rock and roll? Let's go.

To Schedule or Not to Schedule, That Is the Question!

If you haven't heard, most families of twins do not allow their twins to feed on demand but rather have them on a schedule. At this time, you can't even begin to consider a sleep schedule; however, you can start to establish a feeding schedule in the first month. The reason many twin families opt to skip on-demand feeds is because if your babies opt to not feed at the same time, you're going to be feeding one kiddo or the other pretty much around the clock. Let's remember that you need sleep at some point, and you'll need to eat and wash, too.

I know that some parents of twins are very militant about their duo's schedule, but I recommend taking a tiny chill pill here and giving yourself a little wiggle room. If you get too stressed about it, consider getting even wigglier. Just be careful to make sure you are feeding EACH CHILD enough each day. (Yes, you should consider tracking this, too. It's hard to keep on top of it all each day. It really is.)

When my twins were this age, the shine was still on the apple, so to speak. I enjoyed being with them as much as I could, and I'm glad I did. But I tried to stay so tightly on a schedule that it gave me anxiety if we were off even by a little. That's why I'll always recommend that you be a bit "wiggly" with your daily plans, especially in the beginning. When your twins are graduating kindergarten, you're not going to remember the night that they had their last feed thirty minutes late. Keep your mind on the bigger picture and enjoy the moments you have with your tiny duo.

You should note that while the AAP recommends on-demand feeding with singletons, they recommend feeding on a schedule for twins. They also recommend that when one baby eats, the other twin should, too. Yes, even if the other kiddo is sleeping, you should wake them up.

Although I don't suggest that you follow a strict schedule, you *may* see a rhythm appearing in your day. You'll see sleep and brief wake periods happening between each feeding.

For your own printable copy of this schedule, see the QR code.

A few things to note about this schedule:

- It doesn't include naps. That's because sleep is so unpredictable at this age. Your babies might only stay up for forty-five minutes while they are eating before wanting to go back to sleep.
- There are gentle reminders throughout the day to take care of yourself, too. That can mean different things to different people, but be sure that you are taking several moments each day to breathe.

- There are times throughout the day where going out for a walk is suggested. I sincerely encourage you to get out as much as you can. Fresh air is good for you, your twins, and everyone's mental health.
- You'll also want to consider a designated bedtime each night, and it's never too soon to start a bedtime routine. Many folks opt to do a bath before their night feed. This is a great time for everyone to unwind, and since your babies are so tiny (and so slippery), bathing them one at a time is a great opportunity to bond with them individually. This schedule is ideal for a 7:30/8 PM bedtime, but you can be wiggly here.

The Rhythm Is Gonna Get You

True, I'm quoting a 1987 Gloria Estefan song, and it's to make you pay special attention to your children's rhythms. One baby may be a night owl while the other is falling asleep even before you start your bedtime story. Remember, your twins are two different people with the same birthday. Take notice of when each of your children wants to feed, sleep, play, be held, or burp, and when each tends to whine, and you may discover they actually have their own routine. Try, when possible, to follow your kiddos' rhythms, and there will be more peace in your home.

Feeding and Sleep Logging

I know I've mentioned this before, but it's worth repeating: Many parents find it helpful to log their twins' feeding, sleep, and diaper changes at this age. Even if you don't do this every day, a four-day log can be very enlightening. Kim and I recommend also noting the time that they wake each day and the time that they go to sleep for bedtime. Especially as their sleep develops, this will help you determine when you can regularly plan to put them down for the night.

You can download our app using the QR code to keep track of feedings, poops, and more.

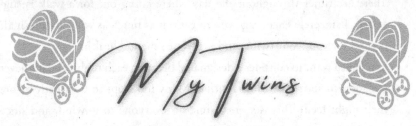

First Month Home
Daily Schedule

Sample Schedule Based on 3hr Feedings*

6am		6pm 🦆
7am 🧷 🍼		7pm 🧷 🍼
8am		8pm
9am ☕		9pm ☕
10am 🧷 🍼		10pm 🧷 🍼
11am 🚼		11pm
12pm		12am
1pm 🧷 🍼		1am 🧷 🍼
2pm		2am
3pm ☕		3am
4pm 🧷 🍼		4am 🧷 🍼
5pm 🚼		5am

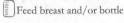Feed breast and/or bottle   Change

Go Outside   Sponge Bath   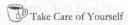Take Care of Yourself

*Always check with your doc about schedule specifics
for your particular twins

Remember to SOAR

 Some parents assume their babies are hungry every time they cry, but when it comes to feeding, it's important to remember to SOAR:

- *Stop* and take a breath so that you are ready to focus and ready to read your babies' cues.
- *Observe* your babies' cries: Over time, you'll hear slight differences that can tip you off to what the issue may be—whether they're hungry or looking for something else.
- *Assess* the situation: When did they last eat? Are they experiencing a growth spurt? How long have they been awake? What's going on in their environment? How long have they been awake? Does their diaper need changing? What else might they be trying to tell you?
- *Respond* with feeding or soothing, as appropriate.

If you constantly respond to crying by feeding your baby without assessing if they might have another need, you may miss the chance to help soothe them in other ways that better match that need.

Should I Wake My Babies to Feed?

There is conflicting advice about waking babies for feeds. Generally, if they haven't eaten in three hours, I say wake them up, but when your babies are discharged from the hospital or during your first doctor's appointment, it's important to ask your doctor this very question.

Most likely your doc will say that they need to eat every three hours, or sometimes even every two, depending on birth weight. There is no wiggle room here. Your doc is the one who has eyes on your babies and knows their weights and any issues. So regardless of what you read online, or hear from a friend, always do what the doc says when it comes to how much your babies need to eat. Please.

Should I Introduce a Bottle Now?

Yes, you should introduce a bottle now. Maybe not today, but definitely within the first month. Some lactation consultants say no bottles under any circumstances until breastfeeding is established, but having two infants rely on you twenty-four hours a day, seven days a week will be overwhelming if you can't ever have someone else feed them. It's tougher to rest or take a nice shower, not to mention leave your house, run to the doctor yourself, or whatever else you choose to do, when you're the human vending machine. Bottles allow someone else to use expressed milk or formula to feed your babies. You may even want to exclusively pump, meaning that you never have a baby to "the tap", and you always used expressed milk. As I said before, there is no wrong way. Whatever works best for you.

I was an exclusive pumper. I had a very hard time getting the twins to latch, and I decided it wasn't worth the struggle. It's one of the reasons I became a CLC. As they say, hindsight is 20/20, and I wish I would have tried to get them to latch more. It would have been good for them and, honestly, even better for me. If I were my own lactation consultant, I would have recommended more skin-to-skin time and more attempts at latching when I was comfortable.

Many families introduce bottles during the first few months anyway, when Mama Bear has to go back to work. It will be an easier transition if you make that introduction now, and you'll always have the ability to either use a bottle or not.

As far as "nipple confusion" goes, I'd like to say, personally *and* professionally, that I wouldn't worry about this. I would, however, stay on a slow/lowest-flow nipple. If your babies are used to drinking from you, they are used to a fairly slow flow because they are setting the pace. With a higher-flow nipple, you can see when you hold the bottle upside down that milk will just spill out; that means your babies don't have as much control. In my opinion, nipple confusion occurs because a baby finds an easier way to do things and starts to prefer that. So, the closer you can stay to the flow of your own body, the less confusion there will be all around.

How Will I Recognize My Babies' Cues?

There are some universal cues that signify hunger in newborns, but because your babies are unique, they'll have their own rhythms, styles of feeding, and ways of communicating. It may not happen overnight, but eventually you will be able to tell right away when they're hungry. For now—since you guys just met, after all—look for things like:

- Licking lips.
- Sticking out the tongue.

- Rooting (moving jaw and mouth or head in search of the breast or bottle).
- Putting hand to mouth repeatedly.
- Opening the mouth.
- Fussiness.
- Sucking on everything around.

Crying is a hunger cue as well, of course. A baby's primal brain encourages them to cry to signal urgent needs. But crying is a late sign of hunger and can make it hard for your babies to settle down to eat, so it's best to watch for hunger cues before crying starts. Learning to recognize your kiddos' early hunger cues will help you respond more quickly to their needs, keeping your twins from getting dysregulated and reducing the need for soothing.

It's important to remember, however, that even sucking does not always mean your babies are hungry. Babies suck not only from hunger but also for comfort, and it can be hard at first for parents to tell the difference. Sometimes, your twins just need to be cuddled or changed.

As your babies' bodies and tummies grow and they are able to eat less frequently, you can use your babies' cues to know the difference between hunger and other needs, and respond accordingly. You'll get the hang of it in no time.

Rooting for You

If one (or both) of your twins are fussing and you are not sure if they are hungry, the rooting reflex is your friend! Put your baby near your breast or the bottle, and stroke their cheek. If they turn toward and root for the breast or bottle, then they *are* hungry. Using this tip in the first several months (until their reflex fades) will help you differentiate your babies' hunger cries so that you know them when you hear them going forward.

Feeding Challenges in the First Month

Addressing feeding challenges can help your twins stay on track with sleep this month. Feeding is an integral part of sleep, particularly at this age.

Breastfeeding Challenges

Breastfeeding doesn't always come easily to moms and babies. If you're having challenges, please know that you are not alone.

Most breastfeeding issues arise within the first two weeks of life and can include tongue tie, lip tie, cheek tie, low milk supply, oversupply of milk, mastitis, and an overall poor latch. Whatever breastfeeding challenge you may encounter, please know that there is almost always a solution. Yes, even with twins. Be sure to seek the advice of a professional lactation consultant at the earliest sign of an issue. You'll want someone who is familiar with working with twins and the challenges that come with having two at a time. A good lactation specialist will listen to your goals and help you discover ways to make them happen.

You're not supposed to know everything. Don't be afraid to ask for help! The newborn stage is such a big time in your parenting life, and you need to ease into it. Having a pro at your side will make everything go smoother.

Access Twiniversity's "Breastfeeding Twins" resources at the QR code.

Allergies

Some babies exhibit allergic reactions to breast milk or formula, such as tummy troubles, skin reactions, or what I like to call spider web poop (trust me, you'll know what I mean if you see it, and it's pretty rare, so don't stress).

If the reaction is to breast milk, usually the baby is reacting not to anything inherent to the milk itself but to a particular food or drink their mother is taking in that is then getting converted into breast milk. Babies' most common allergens are dairy, soy, eggs, corn, and gluten.

If you think one or both of your twinnies might have a food allergy, consult with your pediatrician on next steps. It's helpful to take a picture of any rashes and even those gross poopy diapers. If the doc can see with their own eyes what a rash or poop looks like, they may be able to solve the mystery of what is bothering your twinnies faster. Just remember whose poop is whose and which rash belongs to what baby.

Reflux and GERD

UGH! Can you hear me rolling my eyes from there? Reflux was the BANE OF MY EXISTENCE when my twinnies were born. My Baby A suffered so badly from reflux that I feel like I should have a PhD on this topic alone! Reflux is typically due to an immature digestive system, and because our babies are often born on the earlier side (even two weeks early can make a difference), it's common with newborn twins. Usually, reflux is no cause for concern (though if it's interfering with your babies' growth, then yup, it becomes an issue).

Reflux—often just called spitting up—is common in singleton babies, too; it's reported in 40 to 65 percent of healthy infants. It can have a few different triggers:

- Drinking too quickly.
- Milk or formula flow that is too fast, whether because of an overactive letdown, very full breasts when breastfeeding, or an inappropriate bottle nipple. (A quick FYI here: Bottle nipples come in different "levels." The lower the number, the slower the flow. If you use the wrong level, the milk may come out too quickly!)
- Swallowing a lot of air during the feed.
- Drinking too much (happens more with bottle-fed babies).

Although it may sometimes seem like their entire feed comes back up afterward, looks can be deceiving, and odds are most of it has actually stayed down.

Gastroesophageal reflux disease, or GERD, is different. It shows up when the valve between the esophagus and the stomach allows contents of the stomach to regularly flow up and cause additional problems. It can be a big sleep disruptor! Please check with your pediatrician if you feel that your baby is spitting up significantly after feeding or if you're seeing any of the following behavior:

1. Vomiting after eating.
2. Constant hiccups.
3. Chronic irritability.
4. Discomfort when lying on their back.
5. Chronic cough and/or congestion.
6. Arching of their back after a feeding.
7. An acidic smell to their breath when they cry after a feeding.

There are a few things you can try to help care for your baby if they have GERD:

- Holding them upright for thirty minutes after feeding.
- Feeding them as a start to the day, rather than right before their first nap, and then making sure to keep them upright for thirty minutes of playing before putting them back down to sleep.
- Offering smaller, more frequent feedings.
- Using the alternative tummy time positions we suggested in the "Development" section to avoid additional pressure on their stomach, which may cause additional discomfort.
- Rather than nursing them to sleep, nursing them, burping them, and then holding them upright as they fall asleep.
- Removing dairy from your diet or formula. The AAP says that when a mother drinks cow's milk, small amounts may appear in her breast milk. And several studies have shown that breastfed infants may benefit from their mothers cutting out both cow's milk and eggs.

Babies with GERD often feed for shorter periods of time during the day and then fuss after feeding, though they tend to do a little better with their nighttime feeds—maybe because they are not awake enough to associate feeding with the pain that they experience afterward, or maybe they are just a lot more relaxed and taking in less air with their gulps.

Babies with reflux might hold on to their night feedings a bit longer than other babies—you'll want to work with your pediatrician before weaning them from their night feeding to make sure that they are getting enough nourishment during the day. This is tough because one or both of your babies may want an extra feeding at night to complete their day, yet after they feed, they are lying back down to sleep, which can make reflux worse.

Babies with GERD usually get used to being held to sleep—but don't worry at this stage. It's important to get your baby the nutrients that they need—pain-free—and the sleep that they need any way you can.

If either or one of your babies has very severe reflux, your pediatrician may recommend moving to a medical grade formula or combining it with breast milk to make it easier and quicker for them to digest, so less is likely to come up. There are a lot of solutions you can try before you get to that point, but if you do, know that you can reach out to us at community@Twiniversity.com. We've had a lot of families in that same boat, and speaking to other families who have "been there and done that" can help you emotionally and even financially. Many families have found hacks on how to save on medications and formula for babies with severe GERD.

Breastfeeding a Baby with Reflux

Sometimes moms forget that the position their babies are often in when breastfeeding is pretty flat and therefore more likely to result in reflux. Sometimes the pain in their tiny tummies can make babies with reflux not want any boob time. That doesn't mean your babies are rejecting you or don't want to feed from you. They may just be telling you that the position isn't working because it's making them too uncomfortable.

If you suspect one or both of your twins have reflux, the first thing you can try is feeding them in a position where gravity is on your side. I have moms who lean back on a bed at around a 45-degree angle and place their babies on top of them, with the top of the baby's head pointed toward the ceiling. I have moms who position themselves in a seated position and hold their breastfeeding baby in a football hold, but with their feet at more of an angle so they are as vertical as possible while still retaining a good latch. I've even had moms WALK around and breastfeed with their babies almost in a standing position. If both of your newborns are struggling with reflux, you may want to consider skipping tandem feedings so you can really focus on keeping each baby comfortable while they're feeding.

Personally, I didn't want to have my Baby B latch because my Baby A's reflux meant she couldn't, and I had this horrible guilt that if they *both* didn't latch, then *neither* of them should. I wish someone would have told me it was OK to do what I could, even if it was just with one baby. I've learned a lot the "hard way," as they say, and I don't want you making those same mistakes. So, please: Do what you can. Even if it's just with one baby. You will find time to bond with the other in some other way.

Supplementing with Formula at This Age

You may have heard that supplementing can help your twins sleep for longer stretches, particularly at night. I will never and have never recommended supplementing for only this purpose. Of course, if you have to supplement or want to supplement, you should. I'll say it again so the people in the back can hear: There is no wrong way to feed a baby as long as that baby gets fed! Got it? Good.

 Attachment

Attachment is a deep and durable emotional link that connects you to your children and is created by tuning in to your twins' cues and responding appropriately to their needs. A strong attachment will help your duo feel safe and sleep better both now and in the future. At this stage, you are building basic trust to support this attachment.

A securely attached baby is confident in their caregiver's ability to care for them and in their caregiver's availability: *They may not always be right next to me, but they will come when I call them.* Decades of research show this type of attachment has the best outcomes in a baby's physical, social, emotional, and cognitive development, both in the short and long term.

When it comes to nighttime sleep, quality daytime and nighttime caretaking and availability can add to a secure attachment. This caretaking includes sensitivity to your twins' needs plus appropriate and consistent responses to their cues—some parents choose co-sleeping because it checks these boxes. For more on attachment, please see our introduction to the topic in chapter 1.

Attachment Parenting

Attachment theory (and the concept of attachment) is not the same as *attachment parenting*. There is some overlap, however. Attachment parenting promotes the idea of feeding with love and respect, responding with sensitivity (particularly using touch and babywearing), and providing consistent and loving care. Physically and emotionally safe sleep is also a big tenet, as is striving for a healthy balance between personal and family life.

Is it possible to practice attachment parenting with twins? Yes. As with schedules at this time, you may need to be a little wiggly about your attachment parenting rules, but if you want to give it a try, go for it.

Some of the main components of attachment parenting are co-sleeping (having your babies sleep near you; not to be confused with co-bedding/family bed), babywearing, lots of skin-to-skin time, being responsive to their cries, and breastfeeding. These are all things that are very possible to do with twins. You can't always do all of them with both kids at once, but a partner/family member/helper can assist.

Bonding with Your Twins in the First Month

Some of us feel an intense bond with our babies the minute they're born. For many other parents, that passionate connection isn't immediate—and they feel guilty about it. Be kind to yourself. Not everyone experiences that bond overnight. There is a good chance that your partner may be feeling the same thing. You might want to consider discussing it with them if you are worried about bonding with the babies.

If you don't feel that bond yet, just know that bonding doesn't have to impact attachment. Secure attachment is the result of an *ongoing* process of positive give-and-take. It's about bonding *over time*. Rome wasn't built in a day, people. It's OK to feel like you delivered two little strangers. You'll get to know them, and you'll get to love them over time. There is no rush here.

Bonding with our babies comes from reading their cues, responding to them, and empathizing with their experiences. All of these actions are forms of *parent-infant synchrony*.

Your attachment tasks within the first month are fairly straightforward. Your twins are looking for you to:

- Meet their needs by responding to their cries.
- Meet their needs by feeding them, changing their diapers, putting a roof over their heads, and providing emotional/physical safety.
- Let them regularly hear your voice.
- Make eye contact.
- Exhibit signs of affection.
- Provide nurturing touch.

These first few weeks, you'll spend a lot of time simply giving your babies attention and observing them. In these days of constant multitasking, this quiet time with your newborns may feel a little boring and inactive. If that's how it feels . . . you're doing it right! This is your chance to learn to read your twins' cues and for your kids to learn to read yours.

During this time, we want you to focus on your twins and YOURSELF. Learning your newborns' cues will allow you to respond to their fussiness more quickly and accurately—whether simply to calm them or help them learn to sleep. Your time investment now will pay off with more "me time" . . . and more sleep . . . later.

PUT! DOWN! YOUR! PHONE! Please.

Your twins' bedtime routine, in particular, is one of the greatest opportunities for you to connect and bond with your babies. Leave your phone, tablet, and any other screens out of reach so your focus is fully on snuggling, smooching, and cuddling those sweet babies. If you are distracted by work emails or the latest episode of whatever series you are currently bingeing while they nap, your facial expressions won't be reflective of how you feel toward them. If you're reading a crappy work email, your babies will see your potentially angry expression, and that's not very calming now, is it?

Giving your children your full attention during bedtime, as well as other times of the day, of course, will help you become fully present and will make your babies feel more secure when falling asleep.

Ways to Bond with Your Babies

Here are some of the easiest ways you can nudge attachment along. Some of these may come naturally to you. Others . . . maybe not so much.

Create Routines and Predictability

Routines give your twins something that they can count on. They let your twins learn "I know what's coming next," which is comforting.

While in utero, everything in your twins' world was simple and consistent. They were in a warm environment, fed constantly, and comforted by the soothing sound of their twin's and mom's heartbeats. When your twins are born, they enter a world that is new and unfamiliar, filled with foreign sights, sounds, and smells. Yeah, it can be a bit overwhelming.

We have routines for our days as adults, too. We wake up in the morning and fall asleep at the end of the day, usually at predictable times. We tend to work certain hours and eat around the same times every day. Routines bring structure to our lives, and structure and predictability help us feel secure. Putting routines in place for your twins will do the same and bring about positive benefits for your children and your family as a whole.

You can begin to weave small routines into your days and evenings as early as your twins' first week. Start by practicing a few minutes of tummy time in the morning, reading to them in the afternoon, and maybe giving them a nice warm bath and a massage in the evening before you put them down to bed.

Our goal is to create routines that our babies can expect and count on—and not just at bedtime, mealtime, and bath time. For example, you might have a special toy for diaper changes or a favorite song as you start a daily walk.

Bedtime routines can help your baby fall asleep faster and help diffuse nighttime fussiness. Some babies fall into routines easily, while others may take some time to adjust. Believe it or not, it only takes a week (or less) for most young babies to acclimate to new routines.

Four Areas Where You Can Build Easy Routines with Your Twins

Feeding

Some parents put on some classical music or hum a song while feeding. Others put their babies safely in a bouncer while they go prep everything they need for feeding. Something as simple as that will let your twins know it's almost chow time!

Playtime

Give your twins regular tummy time on the same blanket or play mat. Use this blanket or play mat around the same time every day. Consistency is key!

Naps

Try to do the same two or three things before putting your twins down for each nap. These can be simple and quick, like singing a little lullaby, changing them, and swaddling them.

Bedtime

Establish a few cozy and relaxing steps before putting your twins down for bed. Baths, books, and massage are all wonderful routines you can start early on.

Determine which parts of the routines each twin loves, and include these throughout each day. But remember: Try not to get too caught up with rigid schedules at this time—remain a bit wiggly. Try to set up a nice consistent flow to your day, though. Do things in the same order regularly. It may make you feel like you're in the movie *Groundhog Day* with Bill Murray, but that's a good sign, in all honesty. Babies typically sleep, eat, have a brief period of activity, and then begin to get tired again. You can use this natural cycle as your framework. Observe your children's patterns to determine their natural flow and blend your routines in.

Be Responsive

Respond to your babies' needs promptly. No, you don't need to run; just let them know you heard them and will be there as soon as you can. This is an easy way to build a bond with your twins. If they cry because they are wet, changing them lets them know you've heard them. If they make hungry noises, feeding them teaches them what they need to feel better, and that you can be trusted to help. If you can't address their needs immediately, if possible, talk to them while you finish whatever you're doing (such as taking care of their twin!). You can't spoil a baby by being "too responsive" in the first few months of life.

Hold Them!

Hug your babies, cuddle them, look into their eyes, and when they coo at you, coo back! Don't overlook the power of skin-to-skin contact. Your touch and warmth release the calming chemical oxytocin in your babies' brains, which can bring down stress levels for all of you.

Let the Guilt Go!

If you don't get to hold each of your babies for exactly the same amount of time each day, they aren't going to need more therapy when they are older. Every day, just do the best you can. Don't stress about trying to be "equal"; rather focus on being "fair." If you had a lot of skin-to-skin time with one baby today, try to make an effort to pay a little more attention to your other cutie the next day. Things will NEVER be equal, so let that go now. I've watched parents struggle with this for over a decade now, and I wish we could reset the feelings we have around being twin parents. It's OK to spend more time with one now and then. It's OK to even feel more connected with one than the other at times, though as soon as you realize that's the case, try to balance it out. You won't be able to feel the same connection with the other twin if you don't put in the work.

I'm very out about "twin favoring" when my kids were little. I had one twin that just needed me more, and therefore I bonded with her more in the beginning. It didn't mean I loved her twin brother any less; it just meant that I HAD to spend more time with her because of her medical issues. Her reflux was so bad that it was a real challenge to feed her, and everyone that I had around to help was too afraid to do it. It all fell on me. My dude was easy. He was happy all the time, easy to make laugh—we nicknamed him Frank the Tank because he was like a bottomless pit when it came to bottles.

I knew I was spending more time bonding with my baby girl, and it was eating me from the inside out because I didn't feel that same connection with my son. One day, finally, I talked to my hubs about this, and we made a pact that he would try harder to become the feeding whisperer for my daughter so I could spend more time with my boy.

It worked. All I needed to do was voice my concerns, and we worked it out. If you feel the same way, like you're connecting with one twin more than the other, take a deep breath, tell someone, and see if you can come up with a plan to fix what you think needs fixin'.

Kangaroo Care

Have you heard about *kangaroo care*? We've actually already talked about it using another name: *skin-to-skin*. Kangaroo care is the more traditional name.

A quick detour on why it's called kangaroo care: Baby kangaroos are born premature. The kangaroo has one of the shorter gestation periods in the animal kingdom, between twenty-eight and thirty-three days. When the teeny-tiny underdeveloped kangaroo is born, it is not even an inch long but instinctively knows to travel to its mama's pouch, where it remains gestating for another eight months until it is ready to meet the world.

When my twins were in the NICU it was highly recommended by all the medical practitioners we met that we have kangaroo care time with the twinnies. Basically, because they were six weeks early, they needed to live in our "pouch" for a bit longer. Now, sure, I don't have a pouch, but I could easily unbutton my shirt, remove their tiny undershirt, and lay them flat against my skin. My husband would do the same.

Kangaroo care is the primary reason I tell parents to NOT pack T-shirts or polo shirts in their hospital bag. Only pack shirts that have buttons down the front for easy skin access.

Kangaroo care is particularly helpful with low birth weight or premature babies, since it gives them similar benefits as an incubator (and more, because they are getting touch as well). It's also been shown to stabilize their breathing and heart rate and reduce the risk of infection. But all newborns can benefit from kangaroo care.

For mama bears, regular skin-to-skin contact supports both breastfeeding and bonding because it stimulates the release of helpful hormones, specifically prolactin and oxytocin, from the pituitary gland. It helps initiate breastfeeding earlier, which helps babies gain weight faster. Kangaroo care also helps papa and partner bears develop a close relationship with their babies and increases parental confidence. Your twins know your voice, too. They may not know the exact pitch, because the sound was a little more muffled than mom's while they were in utero, but they know the rhythm of your voice. Trust me, they know it's you, and they love you and want snuggle time with you.

To practice safe kangaroo care, place one or both babies naked (except for diapers for cleanliness and hats to keep their heads warm) in an upright position on your chest. (Yes, you can have both babies on you at once as long as you have another pair of hands ready to assist.) Support them in this position using clothes or other cloth tied around your chest, leaving their heads free and making sure their faces can be seen to allow for unobstructed breathing and for you to read their cues.

 ## Soothing

Part of the attachment and bonding process is the act of soothing your newborns when they cry or get fussy. Eventually, you will learn to read their cues to understand exactly which need they need met, but until then, there are some simple ways to soothe them and help them feel safe and secure.

Soothing is also the first step to getting your babies to sleep at this stage. Remember, an upset and dysregulated kiddo is not calm enough to be lulled to sleep.

Remember when you learned about your babies' current state of brain development? They are operating from the primal brain, and their rage, fear, and separation distress systems are helping them stay safe. It is not surprising that they become afraid after hearing a loud noise or get upset when you put them down after a cozy, warm snuggle. Babies are genetically programmed to cry out for soothing when they are upset. Crying is their way of asking for help in easing frightening emotions and scary-at-times bodily sensations.

The process of crying does not negatively affect a baby's developing brain. What does negatively affect the brain is *prolonged* unsoothed distress, which causes babies to become dysregulated. Your twins learn to self-regulate by experiencing and learning how to handle short periods of frustration and light dysregulation only when these periods are age appropriate and overseen by a supportive parent or caregiver. The problem is that we're often *not told* what is age appropriate and what our babies can handle developmentally (which is why we've included a "Development" section in each chapter of this book). Frustration beyond a baby's developmental capacity leads to withdrawal behavior. This is not the same as independence—it's a coping mechanism. We are not looking for quiet, independent kiddos at this age.

In fact, crying is a good thing. OK, I can hear you laughing right now. Yes, I mean it—crying is a good thing. It's your babies' way of communicating with you. Think of it this way: If you and your BFF have an argument, what's better: talking about it and working it out or getting the silent treatment? Your babies' cries are their version of talking it out. Sure, there will be moments where you just can't take it, and it's totally OK to step away for a moment or two as long as they are in a safe space. But ultimately, your teeny-tiny tots are trying to tell you something when they cry, and it's up to you to figure out what it is.

At this stage, we respond to our infants and soothe them because they are incapable of doing it themselves. This teaches them what it feels like to be soothed and regulated, which in turn helps them learn to self-soothe in the future. As they learn new self-soothing techniques, they will repeat the ones that bring them to the regulated state they have learned to experience with your help.

In other words, soothing is important both to comfort your baby in the moment and to support their healthy brain development for long-term growth and success.

Believe it or not, your continued regular response can keep your twins from exhibiting intense reactions to stress in the future. This comes from building trust. They learn to trust that their communication will be heard. If your baby knows that you'll respond to them in short order, they are less likely to overdo it on the crying or fussiness.

When a baby uses a cue that seems to work—when a caregiver responds to that cue by meeting the correct need—they will repeat it. As you see your own babies' cues repeat, it will get easier for you to recognize their needs. Soon, you will have your own special language with your twins. The more you respond to their cues, the faster they will learn which cues work best. Remember to SOAR! (If you need a refresher, check out page 12.)

Tips for Soothing Your Twinnies

Eventually, your kids will have many tools in their self-soothing toolbox that they can use to soothe themselves. For now, while you're in charge of soothing them, we're giving you a number of soothing tools to add to *your* soothing toolbox. Not every new parent knows how to soothe a baby. I've worked with several parents who didn't know a single soothing technique. And I'd really like to make sure your toolbox is filled.

The key to soothing your twins is knowing about their original home: the womb. There, the environment had a sound level that was to their liking, they were warm and comfortable, and they had access to food when they needed it. Your job is to, as much as possible, replicate this environment to soothe them as they try to make sense of their new world. Sometimes close contact is enough to soothe them, but sometimes they need more. Here are some of the most effective ways to soothe your savage beasts.

Dr. Harvey Karp's popular book *The Happiest Baby on the Block: The New Way to Calm Crying and Help Your Newborn Baby Sleep Longer* recommends what he calls the five Ss: swaddling, side holding, "sh-sh-shing," swinging, and sucking—to get baby through the first few months.

Swaddling

 Swaddling your babies isn't a new thing. There are depictions of babies being swaddled dating as far back as the Paleolithic Era. So yeah, it's been around a minute. Swaddling is tightly wrapping your baby to restrict the movement of their arms and legs. This is especially helpful at this stage due to the Moro, or startle, reflex (see page 47), where their arms and legs can suddenly move involuntarily both when they are awake and asleep.

The pressure of swaddling, similar to what your babies felt in utero, comforts them and can lengthen their sleep—and it often works especially well alongside white noise (more on that shortly).

There are a lot of great swaddling products to choose from. We've compiled a list you can read by using the QR code.

As simple as it may seem, swaddling does come with some risks. There are some safety concerns that every parent should be aware of when swaddling their baby, including suffocation, hip dysplasia, and overheating. However, if swaddling is done properly and safely, most of these risks can be avoided (see the "How to Swaddle Safely" box below).

Please keep in mind that while swaddling babies can be very helpful during sleep, it is not recommended that you swaddle your baby during their wakeful hours, as they need time to move and explore their world and environment.

How to Swaddle Safely

- A baby's legs and hips should not be wrapped so tightly as to completely restrict movement.
- Legs should be free to move up and out.
- Arms are bound firmly but not too tightly (avoid too much pressure on the chest).
- When swaddling your baby for sleep, NEVER lay them down on their stomach. There is a high correlation between suffocation and babies who are swaddled and laid on their tummy to sleep.
- Be aware of their temperature and dress them accordingly—sometimes, just a diaper underneath is sufficient. I generally use the rule that your babies should wear one more layer than you are in your home. So if it's hot in your house, just a diaper and a swaddle is fine. If you're cold and walking around in a sweater, dress them in a onesie and then the swaddle.
- Only swaddle your baby to calm them or for sleeping.
- Swaddling should be discontinued once your baby is rolling or close to doing, so that they don't roll onto their stomach and get stuck, unable to breathe.

BENEFITS OF SWADDLING

If you are safely swaddling your baby, you may see the following benefits:

- Longer and deeper sleep. (Note that this is also a risk factor, as a baby in deep sleep may not awaken if they get themselves into an unsafe sleeping situation.)
- Less crying.
- Easier calming and soothing.

- A newborn that cannot wiggle into dangerous positions in their crib (like getting a leg stuck between the mattress and the railing or between two slats of a crib).
- A reduction in the risk that your baby will roll onto their stomach.
- Less waking due to startling (less arm flailing).

ALTERNATIVES TO SWADDLING

Occasionally, a baby just doesn't like being swaddled. Yup, it happens.

Don't force it; swaddling is not a requirement. First, you can try a modified swaddle, if you have a swaddle blanket that allows you to place their hands on their chest instead of down by their sides. Consider a "half swaddle" that keeps your baby's arms outside of the tightly wrapped blanket. If that doesn't work, you can double down on the other soothing options to help your baby fall asleep, like rocking, walking, breastfeeding, and babywearing (carrying them close to your body with a sling, small carrier, or wrap). Yes, that's a challenge if they BOTH don't want to be swaddled, but Mother Nature is pretty good about this, and odds are, if you have a baby that doesn't like to be swaddled, your other baby will like it just fine.

If you find that both of your twins aren't big fans of the ol' swaddleroonie, then you'll have to work with your partner to divide and conquer for bedtime. If you are flying solo during this time, try your best to comfort them however you safely can.

Side Holding

Some babies find being on their side is very soothing, particularly if they have reflux or other tummy troubles. This is something that the nurses helped me practice with my twins when they were in the NICU. To do this, hold them gently on their side in your arms or on your lap. You can use side holding to soothe them *before* sleep, but remember that there is a difference between holding a baby on their side and putting them to sleep on their side. Holding them on their side is wonderful; side sleeping is dangerous, as they could easily roll onto their face or tummy where their breathing could become obstructed, particularly if they are swaddled. Always remember "back to sleep": Your babies should always sleep on their backs unless you are specifically told otherwise by your twinnies' doctor.

Shushing and White Noise

Sometimes you'll see a mom holding a newborn and gently bouncing up and down while shushing their baby. That calm rhythmic *"sh-sh-sh"* noise might be all it takes to relax your twinnies. The sound mimics that of a mama bear's heartbeat in utero and is really comforting to your tiny duo. A sound or white noise machine can also be very helpful in replicating relaxing sounds for the babes, helping you provide constant sound. Remember, your uterus was like Times Square on New Year's Eve when you were pregnant. There was a lot of noise going on in there. So "quiet" isn't what they are used to. As an added benefit, white noise can also drown out other noises that might either keep your baby from sleeping or startle them awake, like your watching TV in the living room or listening to music while you relax.

Swinging

Gently rocking and swinging our babies to calm them is so instinctive that we rarely have to mention it. But do you know why it works? The gentle motion triggers a calming effect in their brain. It's often an effective way to soothe your newborn.

Many parents of twins find themselves letting their babies nap in a swing, which is why I typically recommend you get at least one of them. Make sure that you follow the directions on your swing to the letter since you want to ensure that you are not creating an unsafe environment for your kiddos. You have to be sure that the swing is age appropriate for your babies, too. Since swings have a scoop shape that can cause a baby's head to fall forward toward their chest and block their airway, it's important to always supervise swing naps so you can reposition their head in an upright position as needed.

Swings are also a great place to safely put one twinnie while you are attending to the other. Often, when I'm working with a new family, an infant swing is my go-to spot for the baby we are not holding at the moment. I could be helping a new parent with a breastfeeding latch while the other twinnie happily rocks right next to us. Swings ROCK! And going back to thinking about re-creating a womb-like environment: Unless you were on very strict bed rest during your pregnancy, your twinnies were used to moving up and down and side to side with your movements as you went about your day. The swing can replicate that movement and relax your babies beautifully.

Sucking

Sucking is a natural part of a baby's self-soothing (see "Newborn Reflexes," page 46), so for parents who are worried that pacifiers are bad or the start of a hard-to-quit habit, take a deep breath. Babies *need* to suck, especially during the first few weeks. It's not just about food; sucking calms a baby's nervous system. Babies who aren't offered pacifiers often suck on their fingers or their hands instead.

You should have a mini arsenal of pacifiers in your home before your babies even get there. Many receive them during baby showers, and if you didn't, grab some ASAP. There will be plenty of times where you literally have to pacify a baby, so pacifiers are going to be a good friend to you.

A Note on Pacifiers

 Pacifiers are commonly used around the world to help babies sleep. And for good reason! They can be an insanely effective tool in your soothing toolbox.

The AAP suggests waiting to use a pacifier until breastfeeding is well established, but then recommends them for both daytime and nighttime sleep because they may also protect babies against sudden infant death syndrome (SIDS). When considering using a pacifier, know that:

- It is a personal choice.
- A pacifier's usefulness is based on your babies' temperaments. If a baby is particularly difficult to soothe, their ability to suck on a pacifier to calm themselves can be especially helpful.
- Pacifiers don't help particularly gassy babies because they tend to swallow more air as they suck.
- If breastfeeding, you'll want to confirm that your babies are latching well, that a pacifier isn't impeding the process, and that the pacifier is being

used appropriately as a tool for soothing, rather than when your babies are hungry.

- You may find that a pacifier is only helpful in particular circumstances (for example, only at night, only during the afternoon when extra soothing is needed, or only at the doctor's office).
- Even if you use a pacifier when your babies sleep, you may choose not to use it when they are awake and fussy, or at least not all the time.
- We suggest not keeping a pacifier in your babies' mouths the majority of the time (babies use their mouths to cue their needs, so it's helpful to allow them to share their current cues and start practicing vocalization that they will use later for more advanced communication).
- Use an age-appropriate pacifier. Yes, they are marked for different ages and stages. As your babies get older and their teeth start to come in, it's important for oral development to make sure that you are using the correct one.

If a baby spits out their pacifier, however, don't automatically replug it! You may be hampering their early attempts to communicate with you and interfering with your ability to differentiate between their cries. Sometimes they will want the pacifier back—and they'll let you know! But if you don't assume it's the pacifier they want, you may realize that they are trying to tell you something else.

Additional Soothing Ideas

Sometimes just looking at your twins and talking to them is helpful. Just knowing that you are there and available to them can calm them down.

We've recommended rocking your babies, but sometimes the obvious step of just picking them up and holding them up on your shoulder can help soothe them. Again, part of what they are looking for is a response from you.

Moving your babies' bodies can also sometimes soothe them. You can try:

- Rolling them on their sides (only when they are awake, of course!).
- Folding their arms and legs in toward their chests (a fetal position might make them feel more like they are back in the womb).

- Gently placing a hand on their chests or tummies.
- Holding them in different positions (some babies prefer to be upright, while others want to snuggle under your arm in a football hold similar to when you might tandem breastfeed them).

You can also try putting them next to their twin. It's amazing how, when new parents arrive home with their twinnies, they seem to put them farther and farther away from each other. Sometimes the simple act of them knowing that their wombmate is there will relax them. If you are having a particularly fussy day, I challenge you to just place them near each other. Then just supervise the awesomeness that is your twins. In my first book, *What to Do When You're Having Two*, I included a diagram on how to co-swaddle your twinnies. You'll be amazed at how relaxed they can become if they are just chilling with their bestie.

When it comes to soothing, you have to try it all. This is not a "one size fits all" kinda thing. You have to embrace trial and error. Try not to get stressed when figuring out the best ways to soothe your twins. If you get stressed, and they are stressed, you're gonna be in quite a pickle. So "fake it till ya make it" and keep trying different soothing techniques until you find the ones that work best for each of your kiddos.

Learn Your Twins' Soothing Cues

OK, this is probably obvious, but crying is a cue that one or both of your babies are upset and need soothing. But as you start to observe them, you will see that they express themselves in ways other than just crying to let you know their needs.

Your babies have two main cues as to their state of regulation that they will give you during this time.

Toward the end of this month, your babies might present their first main cue: a relaxed open face with a smile and wide eyes. This lets you know they are comfortable and want to interact with you.

The second is looking away from you with glazed eyes or a frown or arching away from you with a stiff body. This means they have had enough or would like something different. Your babies are unable to move themselves or even understand why they don't like a particular situation. Neither of your babies can limit their own stimulation, so this may be their way of telling you that they would like you to do it for them. Thankfully, the brain of the postpartum mother and baby caregiver is particularly wired to tune in to and recognize these cues. This is your chance to SOAR and determine if they are overstimulated.

Some additional cues you may notice when your baby needs soothing or calming include:

- A "cry face" or a frown.
- Excessive squirming or arching their back.
- Bracing their legs against you or their crib.

Soothing Challenges in the First Month

There are several soothing challenges that you might encounter this month with your twins. Here are a few.

Soothing Colic

According to the Mayo Clinic, colic is "frequent, prolonged and intense crying or fussiness in a healthy infant." Dr. Maryanne Tranter, an expert pediatric nurse practitioner and researcher, shares that it appears in babies under five months with no known cause, and it often occurs in the evening or toward the end of the day, which can set you up for difficulty getting your baby down for the night. If your baby or babies have colic, it can be *very* frustrating to try to soothe them because they appear to be fussy for no clear reason.

Colic is a symptom. Like a fever, it is caused by something else going on with your child. In a lot of cases, a baby is given the diagnosis of colic because the practitioner isn't sure what else is going on.

To be clear, all babies start to use crying as a form of communication at the end of their first month—this is expected, as you learned in the development section. Not all crying is colic. Typically, colic appears around two weeks and lasts through week six or nine—the same time that your babies' brains are starting to mature and are able to manage their sensory overload. They may be starting to smile and coo and engage with the world in a more calm, happy way. If your babies are crying all the time, your fussy babies may just need you to hold them, sit with them calmly, and know that they'll be OK.

When we talk about a baby who has colic, we are referring to a baby who cries significantly *more* than other babies and has no obvious illness or other cause for crying.

TREATABLE CAUSES OF COLIC

While some doctors say you have to just "ride it out" when your baby has colic, the pediatricians we've worked with have found that it sometimes has specific treatable causes. According to Dr. Tranter, colic can be the symptom of three conditions:

1. Tongue and lip ties. A tongue and/or lip tie affects latching, and as a result, babies can take a lot of air into their system while feeding, causing an uncomfortable stomach. They can also end up particularly frustrated and upset because of feeding difficulty.

2. Reflux (particularly silent reflux). The discomfort associated with reflux, or when a baby's stomach muscle pushes the breast milk or formula they drink back up, is a major cause of colic. You can tell when your baby is suffering from reflux because they'll arch their back rigidly in pain and you might even smell that their breath is a bit acidic. For more on reflux, see page 61.

3. Food allergies or intolerances. Your babies might be reacting to something in their formula or something mom ate. Soy and cow milk are the most common issues.

If you feel like one or both of your babies are particularly upset and crying excessively, check with your pediatrician to make sure that these conditions aren't present. For food sensitivities, there are formulas you can try for sensitive tummies, and you may want to keep track of what you are eating to see if there is any direct correlation. I've worked with a few moms who've had to completely eliminate dairy from their own diet since they were breastfeeding, for example.

The issue might also be something else altogether. I suppose to get even with me, my very own Baby A had some pretty significant colic. It was a 9 (out of 10) on the torture scale for us. When traditional treatments didn't help (her doc first recommended gripe water, a specifically formulated solution of different herbs and sodium bicarbonate that you can find at almost any drug store), we dug deeper and found out that the issue was a bit more serious and involved her GI tract. After figuring that out and getting it taken care of, she was one of the happiest babies you'd ever meet.

This is another time I'm going to remind you to go with your gut here. If you suspect something is up with one or both of your babies, keep digging. Maybe even reach out to us here at Twiniversity.

The Witching Hours

Everyone gets to a point in the day where they are just worn out. For most of us, it's typically around 3 PM. We might get a little cranky or grab that next cup of coffee or a slice of something sweet. Well, your twinnies experience a similar struggle.

Your twins are trying to process a whole new world, which can be overwhelming. So, you can expect things to get a little hairy from 3 to 7 PM, which I call the witching hours. By 3 PM, your tiny little babies have already had a huge day. They've seen a lot, heard a lot, smelled a lot, and felt a lot. No wonder they are breaking down! It's no surprise that by late afternoon they are overstimulated and need some downtime. Their witching hour is their breaking point—time to reset. And gang, be warned, they might hit that breaking point at the same time—or they might not.

Preventing overstimulation makes your newborns easier to soothe, and a soothed, calm baby is easier to put to sleep. Limiting stimulation also keeps your babies from habituating, which you learned about in the development section. We want your duo to nap and wake rested rather than come out of a habituated state cranky and in need of more sleep.

Kim's 3 PM Rule

To avoid overstimulation, Kim recommends to families she coaches that, starting at 3 PM, they:

- Turn off the television if it's on.
- Dim the lights a bit.
- Play some calming music.
- Give the twins some time in their swings.

- Grab those pacifiers so they can soothe themselves by sucking.
- Create a routine for other family members who may be coming home at that time to keep the vibe chill.
- If needed (for example, if you have older children with homework or other activities to do), take the twins into another (calmer and quieter) room.

Doing even *one* of these can make your life a lot more peaceful. Think about how you behave during this time of day, and see what changes you can make to your own life to help you during this time. Kim and I also always recommend that if you don't have access to an unlimited supply of help, you might want to focus on at least getting those late afternoon hours covered as often as possible.

 ## Temperament

Remember how I've said that you need to always keep in mind that your twins are two different babies born on the same day? And how they might not have anything in common? Well, when it comes to temperament, it's extra important. Every baby reacts to the world differently. No two humans experience the same thing the same way, and your duo is no different. Yes, even if they are identical. Just because they share 100 percent of the same genes, it doesn't necessarily mean they experience the world in the same way, or react to it in the same way, either.

You might need to prepare your twins for sleep differently according to their particular temperaments. That's the way it goes with a duo. Even with identical twins, you're not guaranteed two babies with the same temperament. You'll also care for them differently when they wake up during the night if they have different temperaments. Yes, this may be a lot to manage, but you can do it. We've helped many families with this issue, and we'll help you figure it out, too.

Read Your Twinnies' Cues

I remember feeling so absolutely overwhelmed when my twins were little. I had two babies with very, very different temperaments. I had one baby, my daughter (Baby A), who got overwhelmed by almost anything, while my other baby, my son (Baby B), wasn't bothered by anything. There were days I felt so guilty that I was giving her all my attention. At the end of the day, I always felt like I hadn't spent enough time with him. But in hindsight, he needed much less. He was easy to soothe, while she was a tiny dumpster fire at times. I was laughing as I wrote that, but it's true. There were days that she was utterly impossible, while my son just played with his feet and giggled. Mother Nature was kind to me. She balanced out my twinnies well. But we have plenty of Twiniversity families whose babies are both as difficult as my daughter.

Spending a lot of time with your two is how you will learn their cues and how to best respond to them, according to their unique temperaments. It can be hard at first! Your twins are not used to all the sights, sounds, and smells around them at first. They may not understand what they feel inside their own tiny bodies. They can't tell you exactly what is making them uncomfortable. All of that is tough for them, and it's tough for you. Luckily, as they mature, they will get better at showing you what they need.

You WILL get the hang of figuring out your duo—even if your twins are both as challenging as my daughter was. Perhaps you'll realize, toward the end of this month, that every time your Baby A fusses and you try to feed them, they don't eat well. They only eat well when they're already soothed. This is a big "aha" for your SOAR (Stop, Observe, Assess, Respond) process. You can check "feeding" off the list as the way to soothe them—even if they're hungry.

Supporting Your Alert Baby or Babies

My Baby A was what Kim calls an alert baby—one who is keenly aware of their surroundings, active, intense, and/or highly sensitive both to internal and external stimuli. Often, alert babies are more difficult to read. It's hard to tell if they are "saying" they are hungry, tired, or in need of a diaper change. They can also be more sensitive to transition.

It's not uncommon to find yourself the parent of an alert baby. In fact, within our Twiniversity team, we found that most of us had an alert baby, or at least one who was more alert than the other, as part of our twin set. Perhaps it's easier for twin parents to see alert baby traits since we have two babies right next to each other.

Parents of alert babies need to be even more responsive to their baby's cues and go even slower (with everything—your feeding, routines, transitions, etc.). Your alert baby's reactions show you not only what they would *like* but also what they *need*.

Sleep can be particularly challenging for alert babies, so know that you'll need to give them extra soothing and that the process of getting them to sleep and teaching them to sleep might take longer. I'm scrunching up my face writing that. I know it's probably what you didn't want to hear, but I'd rather just rip off that bandage and be as honest with you as I can. And as I said, many of us on Twiniversity team had alert babies. If we made it through, so can you. We promise. While sleep coaching can be more difficult for alert babies, it isn't impossible once you've recognized that they have their own rules about how and when they get sleep.

Tips for Alert Newborn Twins

- We've noticed that it can be harder to read the sleep cues of a highly alert baby. They are so engaged in the world that they don't show their cues as clearly, and they sometimes don't become clear until they are overtired. For example, they might not rub their eyes, but their eyes might appear glassy instead. The signs that they are sleepy might only appear once you have gotten into your before-bed sleep routine (which is why it's helpful to have a sense of when your baby usually gets tired and start the routine to lead up to this time).

- Alert newborns may be easier to soothe (and feed) in a separate room, away from the excitement. Their twin, the dog, and the birds outside the window can all easily become distractions for an alert baby.

- Gentle massage works very well for alert newborns, while anything remotely stimulating might be too intense for them at bedtime.

- You may find that your alert baby does not sleep on the go. They are too busy drinking in the outside world. Or you might find they can in the first month or so but not later. Respect that need, and work with them—you can't "train" them to sleep in bright light and noise nor *should* you. It's like suggesting that a natural night owl can easily become a morning person or a coffee drinker can switch to tea and like it. Blasphemy! #coffeerules

You may need to arrange your schedule to allow your alert baby (or babies) to take their naps at home in a consistent location (or at least in the dark with quiet).

The most important thing to understand when caring for your alert baby (or babies) is that some of this book's suggestions won't work *immediately*. You're in a more challenging situation than the parents down the block whose baby starts sleeping through the night on her own at three months (yes, that happens, too). Your job will be a little bit tougher. And with that, it's also important to know that YOU are not doing anything wrong.

In the coming chapters, we'll help you better understand what makes your alert baby (or babies) special so that you can effectively apply the alert baby tips we share with you. And don't stress—even alert babies learn to sleep! I know this personally *and* professionally. It may take a smidgen longer, and you may have to use a more gentle, sensitive approach, but it is totally doable!

It's Not You. It's Them.

Your babies' temperaments may not be what you thought they would be, and it's OK—it's something we just have to accept. Sometimes new parents of twins are looking for the receipt in their hospital bag so they can return them, but having some moments of panic and regret isn't that uncommon for any new mom or dad. Heck, it's not even that uncommon for moms and dads of teens!

You'll have both high and low points, and in the beginning, you may feel like caring for your twins is a little (or a lot) more than you bargained for. You may even feel a little trapped. If that's the case, please make sure that you are keeping an open line of communication with those you trust and telling them how you feel. Parenting can be overwhelming, especially if you have twins that have unpredictable temperaments. Trust us, it's not you. You're doing great. It can be bumpy in the beginning, but you will get the hang of it. You'll get to know your twins like the back of your hand and soon you'll realize that you're having more good moments than stressful ones—and that parenting your duo is a piece of cake.

Getting You and Your Duo to Sleep

Drumroll, please! Yup, the moment you've all been waiting for. Boys and girls, children of all ages, it's time to get those tiny puppies of yours to sleep.

We've set the foundation with solid feeding, attachment, soothing, and you know about temperament. Finally, we can talk about your twinnies' sleep at this age and other ways to support it.

It takes a lot of energy for babies to be awake, take in their new surroundings, and grow both physically and cognitively. Sleep is how they restore themselves. Being a brand-new human is TOUGH! There is so much to learn. I do not envy them, but they have you—they are in great hands.

Eventually, we will want your twinnies to fall asleep on their own, but at this stage, they still need your help quite a bit. Your job is to help them learn the process!

Realistic Expectations

I'd like you to understand what your twins are currently experiencing, sleep-wise, so you know what they are capable of and how to help them meet their needs.

During the first six to eight weeks, their sleep cycle is very unorganized. This means that they will not sleep and wake at standard times each day and night on their own without your guidance. Your duo's sleep will develop in a specific order:

- The morning nap begins to develop around twelve weeks.
- The afternoon nap begins to develop around sixteen weeks.

These developments all occur *around* a certain time, but there is never an exact date, and you have to take your babies' gestational age into consideration here. Also, naps can and often do develop even later than these averages, so don't freak out if you get to sixteen weeks and find your twins still don't nap well, even in the morning.

So long as your babies' sleep/wake cycles remain underdeveloped, don't expect them to sleep for long stretches at a time either overnight or during naps. It's just not in the cards for them at this point. Also, don't worry about creating bad habits. Example: If you find that you are holding one or the other for naps all the time, it's OK. Your twins need you to soothe them to and back to sleep right now no matter how it happens.

It's very common for parents to try a number of different ways to soothe their babies during this stage. You'll hear stories of families going as far as driving their twins around the block to get them to fall asleep. Do what you can at this point. I don't want to sound overly dramatic, but just "get through." The transition from no babies to two babies can be a rocky one. The first month you are all still learning how to deal with each other, so don't put too much pressure on yourself.

Sleep Needs in Healthy Full-Term Babies

There are wide ranges of time given for how much an infant should sleep within a twenty-four-hour period, but the most important finding in infant sleep research in the last fifteen years is that sleep needs can vary widely between babies.

Newborns between zero and three months sleep between ***fourteen and seventeen hours during each twenty-four-hour period***. This total includes both daytime naps and nighttime sleep. Most newborns can only stay awake for about an hour (or an hour and a half maximum) before becoming overtired.

The size of this range can be one of the biggest challenges for twin families. It's possible to have one twin that sleeps fourteen hours a day and another that sleeps seventeen! It's important to not compare one baby to the other, or your twins to your neighbor's kids. There is no typical newborn sleep schedule for babies under six months.

Your goal as a new parent is to help your twins get sleep within this healthy range. Our goal is to give you tips and tricks to help you do this. But it is essential to have realistic expectations. During this time, your babies will sleep in short spurts around the clock. They will need to feed often throughout both the day and night. At this stage, there is not much predictability to sleep patterns or lengths. I recommend you focus on the feeding schedule first and foremost. Your twins will need to eat every three hours (from top of the hour to top of the hour) around the clock. Their sleep will fall into place from there.

What the Heck Are Sleep States?

Interestingly, during the first few months of your twins' lives, their sleep states are similar to the ones they experienced in utero. Their sleep is equally divided between two different states, active (or REM) sleep and deep (or non-REM) sleep. Let's break down what each sleep state is all about so you can better understand your twins' sleep overall.

Active Sleep (REM Sleep)

In the first twenty to thirty minutes of sleep, your babies are in an active state of sleep. This phase is sometimes referred to as "light" sleep and consists of rapid eye movement (REM) sleep.

In active sleep, your baby is mentally digesting and storing all their experiences throughout the day—which plays a critical role in brain development. Blood is flowing to their tiny brains, transporting nutrients to active brain cells.

During active sleep, you can observe rapid eye movement under their closed eyelids. Other characteristics your infants will display during this type of sleep are:

- Irregular breathing.
- Facial expressions (grimacing, puckering of lips, opening/closing mouth, and/or frowning).
- Sucking and other body movements (twitching, startling, stretching).
- Vocalization (whimpering, crying out, whining, grunting), particularly at night.
- Easily startling or awakening.

Easily Awakened During Active Sleep

Do your twins wake as soon as you lay them down? It is very common for young babies to wake easily during the twenty to thirty minutes before they transition into a deeper sleep. Try waiting until your newborns' bodies and eyes are still to put them down. When they are in a deep sleep, they are more likely to stay asleep when they are laid down.

Deep Sleep (Non-REM Sleep)

After active sleep, your twins will move to deep sleep, also sometimes called "quiet" sleep. Again, this stage lasts about twenty to thirty minutes.

During deep sleep, your babies are very still, with eyes closed, rhythmic breaths, and very little muscle movement. Many parents check frequently during this phase to make sure their baby is breathing! Quiet sleep is restorative, allowing the brain to rest.

One of the ways I would check to see if my twins were in a deep (versus active) sleep was to check for "limp limbs." It always made me think of professional wrestling. If you've ever watched a match, the way a person wins is by pinning their opponent as the referee taps the mat for a "1 . . . 2 . . . 3" count. Sometimes the ref will also pick up the arm of the loser, and you'll see it floppily drop to the mat. When my twins were in a deep sleep, I would pick up a tiny hand, raise it slightly, and drop it gently while whispering "1 . . . 2 . . . 3." We aren't a big professional wrestling family now, but my dad and I never missed a WrestleMania when I was in grad school. So, pretending my kids were tiny athletes made me laugh every time. It's how my twins got the nicknames Anaconda (her name is Anna) and Johnstrosity (his name is John)! Those were their baby wrestling names, and I would call them that to entertain myself.

Here are the characteristics of deep sleep:

- Closed eyes with no rapid eye movement.
- Regular, shallow breathing.
- A still, quiet body.
- No spontaneous movement (though your baby may startle, they will remain asleep).

In a deep sleep, your baby may be able to selectively tune out sounds and bright lights and is difficult to awaken. Try not to wake them up or interact with them at this time.

Supporting Your Twins' Sleep

The first month of your twinnies' lives is not the time to start sleep coaching. Even something as simple as putting your baby down to sleep "drowsy but awake," a common sleep coaching step, is not the best idea at this age. A recent study found that starting the drowsy but awake practice at three weeks had *no* effect on a baby's sleep once they reached six months of age. Your babies may be able to naturally put themselves to sleep if they are a bit drowsy, but don't worry if they aren't able to. It's perfectly natural for them to need your help at this point, and again, you are not creating any bad habits.

We'll teach you more about Kim's gentle Baby-Led Sleep Coaching in future months. We've got ya covered!

Sleep Crutches?

Have you heard someone refer to their baby as having a *sleep crutch*? A sleep crutch is what folks refer to as a *negative sleep association*—anything that *has to be done* to or for a baby for them to fall asleep and go back to sleep that they can't do independently. Some examples of sleep crutches are:

- Nursing to sleep.
- Rocking to sleep.
- Replugging their pacifier (which they won't be able to do themselves until at least six months).
- Having them fall asleep in a moving stroller or in the car.
- A combination of several of these.

At this age, almost all babies have at least one sleep crutch. It's expected because they haven't learned how to fall asleep on their own yet. Maybe you rock one of them to sleep with white noise on in the background, and the other cannot fall asleep without their pacifier. We're going to discuss different ways in the next few months to help wean your kiddos off their sleep crutches. For now, don't worry about them.

Your Twinnies' Internal Clocks

When your twinnies are born, they have no internal clock—the hormonal cues that tell them when to be asleep and when to be awake, also known as circadian rhythms. Their circadian rhythms don't become fully mature until around six months, and until they do, your babies just don't have a good sense of whether it is daytime or nighttime. They have no idea if it's nap time or awake time, either. Brand-new twinnies (like during the first week) will just sleep whenever. They will open their eyes for a bit, eat, and go right back to sleep. Honestly, this sounds like my dream life. Who's with me?

What this means is that, at this point in their short life, you are your twins' external clock. You can help them learn when it's time to sleep and when it's time to be awake with light cues and social cues. Eventually, dimming the lights and slowing down the activity around them will give their brain the message that it's time to slow down. Around the third or fourth month, their brain will then secrete the hormone melatonin that will make them drowsy.

Avoid Day/Night Confusion

Often, newborns' days and nights will be totally mixed up. This means they will probably sleep during the day and be wide awake at night. Helping your twinnies learn the difference between day and night is one of the big goals for your first month, and now is a good time to start creating routines that will help them differentiate. Keeping daytime upbeat, bright, and active will be a nice opposition to relaxed, dim, and super chill evening/nighttime. By setting up your day to avoid day/night confusion, you create a solid sleep foundation for the months ahead.

Here are some actions you can take to help your kiddos start to distinguish between night and day:

- Make sure your twins are eating regularly throughout the day. Do not let them sleep longer than three hours. (And remember, when one baby wakes up to eat, wake the other one to eat, too!)
- Expose them to bright outdoor light during the day. If you can't get out of the house, open up all the blinds and curtains and let that sunshine in!
- Keep nighttime activities, like feedings, in dim light and focused. No playtime during the dark/night hours.

Fill the Daytime Sleep Tank

At this age, there is one big thing you can do to make sure your twins are getting enough sleep within each twenty-four-hour period, and that is to make sure they get the sleep they need during the day. We call this *filling your babies' daytime sleep tanks*. And I suggest you fill your twins' daytime sleep tanks any way you can. You can hold them, feed them to sleep, rock them to sleep, whatever they need—just get them to sleep. Contrary to popular belief, the better a baby sleeps during the day, the better they will *also* sleep at night. When they become overtired, their body secretes cortisol, which wakes them up. They might end up waking more frequently at night and earlier in the morning before they are truly rested.

Create a Consistent Bedtime Routine

It's never too early to start thinking about creating an official bedtime routine. This routine can be as simple (or as complicated) as you make it. Some items in a typical nighttime routine are:

- Bath time.
- Story time.
- Massage time.
- Song time.
- Snuggle time.
- Bottle/boob time.

The big key to creating a night routine is consistency. Try to create a routine that is easily replicated. If you start with a bath and end with a bottle in a dimly lit room, do the same each night.

Our bedtime routine was the same day in and day out with my twinnies. Usually, I had an extra pair of hands at this time. Either my mom, my mother-in-law, or my sister was around. We started around 5:30 PM with a bath. I took my time and bathed them one at a time in the kitchen sink. (I always opted for the sink since it forced me to have it empty and ready for bath time.) I'd typically start with my daughter, and I created a little song for her. I used to call her "Floopia" when she was in the tub. The song went like this: "She's Floopia, the littlest mermaid who doesn't live in the sea. She's Floopia, the littlest mermaid who lives in a cup of iced tea." There is no rhyme or reason for that song, but if you start singing it these days, my teenage daughter will finish the lyrics. I inadvertently created a really special memory just by being consistent.

After bath time, we'd usually do a little infant massage. I'm no infant massage specialist, so I'd just rub their tiny toes all the way up to the top of their heads with some delicious-smelling lotion. Then, after I popped them into some fresh pajamas, it was time for a bottle. I'd have some "Classical Baby" music on in the background while they ate. After their bottles, I held them upright for twenty minutes and then placed them calmly in their crib. (My twins did share a crib and slept head-to-head, but please see page 34 for the full story.) I'd stand next to their crib with just the light coming in from the hallway and tell them a story. After the story, I told them I loved them, and they usually were pretty peaceful for a bit after that. I think the massage did 'em in.

I basically kept that same routine, with minor tweaks, through about second grade. When they weren't infants anymore, we skipped the full body massage, but I always did their backs and their hands. If you get into a good system, keep it up! One of the important things I realized when my kiddos were little was that they were also pretty consistent, timing-wise, with their sleep cues. I'm not sure which came first. Was it my sleep routine that guided their sleep cues, or was it the other way around?

At first, you may time this routine for *your* bedtime. But as you start seeing a pattern in your babies' sleep cues, keep an eye out for a time that starts to make sense as *their* bedtime. However, this can be trickier for twins than singletons. With one baby, you can simply follow that baby's cues. With two, you may need to plan a bit differently, especially if one baby has a greater sleep need than the other. If that's the case, you may want to start and finish an entire sleep routine with your sleepier baby and then repeat with the other. You'll honestly have to play this by ear. This is why it's great to start your sleep routine with another adult around if possible. That way each of you can focus on one baby instead of having one adult have to manage both at the same time. If you are flying solo, however, you'll figure out your own system in no time.

During month two, you'll start to ever so slightly regulate your babies' bedtime so that it comes at approximately the same time each evening, within about a thirty-minute window. If it doesn't start moving earlier naturally, in a few months we will guide you through how to move it forward gently over the course of a few nights. Having a familiar bedtime routine will help make this process easier, because your twins will find the process predictable even when it starts a bit earlier.

Naps also benefit from a pre-sleep routine. In this first month (and sometimes until month three or four, depending on temperament), many babies can nap in a bassinet or twin play yard in the living room, in a swing, or even on the go. Enjoy this flexibility while it is here! But it's still helpful to use a routine before each nap, too, though it can be much shorter and just involve feeding or rocking.

Schedule Their Wake-Up Call

Toward the end of this month, you may notice your babies are beginning to wake around the same time each morning. Look for patterns. Perhaps they usually feed at 5 AM and 7:30 AM but don't easily drift back to sleep after their 7:30 AM feeding. They may be trying to tell you that their wake time is 7:30 AM. You can start the day at that time even though you know that their first nap will start soon after that wake-up.

If you do not yet see a pattern, that's OK! It will come—perhaps in a few weeks. If your log notes that your babies' wake times remain particularly inconsistent, for example, 7 AM one day and 9 AM the next, you may decide to simply pick a time to start the day and try that out consistently for a week or so. A regular start time will help start to organize your babies' naps during the day, which will then help you determine when to start their bedtime routine in the evening.

One Early Riser, One Night Owl

Because your twins may have different temperaments, you may notice that one loves waking up early while the other wants to rock all night. There are two ways you can go with this.

Roll with It

You can embrace each of your twins' sleep styles and use the times only one wants to sleep as an opportunity to chill with the other. If you have a baby that wakes up earlier than the other, go liberate them while the other kiddo sleeps a bit longer. Remember, this month, you just need to make it through as happily as possible.

Stay on Schedule

Not all parents are into going with the flow and embracing an early bird or night owl. You can also keep your twins on the same schedule and wake the other if one wakes.

Neither of these are right or wrong. This month you might even do a combo of these. You'll have to feel it out and see what works best for you and your family.

Create a Sleep-Friendly Environment

It is important to create a sleep-inducing environment for your newborns, particularly for night sleep. For more detailed suggestions, check out page 30.

Your babies' sleep environment is important. We shouldn't be trying to "teach" them how to sleep in noise or bright light; it can lead to overstimulation, which can in turn lead to habituation rather than restful sleep. As you've learned, your babies' temperaments are also factors; some babies are naturally more sensitive to their environment than others. But all babies benefit from an environment that supports sleep. Swaddling, white noise, and a dimly lit environment will help your twins sleep easier.

Learn the Sleepy Time Cues

Your newborns will give you cues that say "I'm getting sleepy." Because your newborns will not have a regular sleep schedule at this time—you'll want to put them to sleep whenever they seem drowsy—it's very helpful to learn to recognize these cues. In addition to generally becoming quieter, your babies may show:

- Decreased activity.
- Slower motions.
- Weaker or slower sucking while feeding.
- Disinterest in their surroundings.
- A less focused gaze.
- Drooping eyelids.
- Irregular breathing.
- Yawning. (To avoid a meltdown, try to put them down after the first yawn!)

Crying can be a sign that you've missed some sleep cues and your babies have become overtired, which means they'll be tougher to soothe to sleep. This is why we encourage you to get out your magnifying glass and see if they are trying to communicate their drowsiness to you in some other way—*before* the crying starts.

Drowsiness serves as a transition both into and out of sleep. If left alone, a drowsy baby may go to sleep or may instead gradually awaken. If they have been up for a while (more than an hour) when you start to see these cues, this would be a good time to put them down to sleep.

Sleep Challenges at This Age

It may seem that everything involving sleep is a challenge at this age. Fear not! Things will get easier. In the meantime, there are some aspects of your babies' sleep that might be more of a challenge than they need to be.

The Elements of Baby-Led Sleep Shaping (Month One)

1. Create a sleep-friendly environment for your duo, which should include:
   - Room-darkening shades.
   - Soothing colors.
   - White noise.
   - Cool temperature.

2. Create daily routines:
   - At bedtime, use a consistent, soothing routine. Do this in your twins' nursery if you plan to eventually transition them there, even if you are currently room sharing.
   - Create a shorter pre-nap version of your before-bed routine.
3. Prevent overstimulation by following Kim's 3 PM Rule.
4. Don't let your twins sleep through daytime feedings (i.e., over three hours at a time).
5. Have each twin's last nap end one hour to ninety minutes before their bedtime.

Recognizing When Your Baby Is Habituating

A quick refresher on habituation: Habituation is a soothing mechanism that your twinnies have as newborns that allows them to filter out the "white noise" of life, so to speak, by falling into a dreamlike state. (Aren't babies amazing?) Don't be fooled, though. While habituation looks like sleeping, your babies are using an enormous amount of energy to tune out all the surrounding stimulation.

Why is this important in terms of sleep? Well, you might look at your babies and see that their arms and legs are pulled in and their eyes are closed, and you might think that your babies' sleep tanks are being filled when they aren't. If your kiddos seem cranky after you spent the whole day at a backyard barbecue where they seemed like they slept great, it may all be a ruse! They might "wake up" and be fussy, inconsolable, and utterly exhausted instead of waking up refreshed, as they would if they were truly sleeping.

The newborn skill of habituating is short lived. It begins to wane slowly after eight weeks. By two to three months of age, few infants can still shut down, and almost none can shut off completely when overstimulated. But it's still valuable to learn the signs because, if it happens regularly over a few days, it can lead to fussy feedings and shorter naps. Babies who regularly practice habituation may seem jittery or anxious when awake and can cry easily and often from exhaustion. They will often wake crying and find it difficult to settle down even after feeding.

Keep your eye out for the warning signals that lead to habituation and learn what overstimulates one or both of your babies. Some kiddos have a low tolerance for stimulation and are even more sensitive to environmental disruptions. This temperament will make them more likely to habituate.

How to Recognize Habituation in Your Babies

- Pulling in their arms and legs and closing their eyes.
- What looks like deep sleep in brightly lit and loud surroundings.

Sometimes, no matter how much you try or do, one or both your kiddos just won't chill. You can stand there shushing them, rocking them, and trying to feed them, and they just can't relax. If you find yourself in this situation, you need to evaluate your environment. Is it too bright? Too loud? A new space? All of the above? Strongly consider changing your surroundings. Move into a quiet, dimly lit room and try soothing them there to see what happens. You might find that this was JUST the trick to bring them down from that crying fit—and prevent habituation. Your babies may be trying to say, "Guys, it's just too much."

How to Prevent or Recover from Habituation

- Move to a dim, quiet location.
- After habituating, soothe them before trying to put them back to sleep.
- Prioritize calming your twins' environment and filling their daytime sleep tanks. That may sometimes mean staying home and having a day of quiet and relaxation for everyone.

Premature Birth

If your babies are born before thirty-seven weeks, they are technically considered premature. Perhaps unsurprisingly, there are a few important differences in how we approach sleep for these tiny tots.

If you haven't already, check out the section on adjusted age on page 16. Your babies' adjusted age will help you understand their development and guide your expectations for their sleep.

SENSORY DIFFICULTIES

We all comprehend the world through our senses. We see, hear, and touch things. We experience gravity, and we use our bodies to move. The term *sensory processing* refers to how we integrate the messages coming from the environment and from inside our bodies—a neurological process most of us do automatically and more and more efficiently as we mature—to feel, think, and behave in proportion to what's happening inside and around us.

Children born prematurely are at increased risk for sensory-based issues in which they can either seek more sensory input or get easily overwhelmed by too much of it. Partly because of this, some hospitals have a special preemie discharge plan. You may be given the contact number or email of your delivering hospital's social worker and even be told to consider an evaluation by a professional if you suspect either or both of your twins have any issues. Preemies with sensory difficulties may experience things like being rocked as frightening. Sometimes the sound of a lullaby may be uncomfortable to the ears, and a flickering fluorescent light may look like a strobe light to them. Sensory issues can be at fault for a lot of your premature twinnies' crying.

What seems typical to us can easily overwhelm a child with sensory issues, and this is especially true for preemies, whose brains and bodies are not yet fully developed and able to handle the barrage of sensory input from the world. I'll stand up proudly and say that one of my twins had a *significant* sensory issue for the first few years of his life. I WISH I had known this sleep fact then. It would have saved me a lot of frustration. We had to figure it out the hard way!

My kiddo was a "sensory seeker." Loud music or lights didn't frighten him; it was what he craved. Instead of having to go into a quiet room to soothe my tiny twinnie, I had to put the music up loud and put him directly into sunlight or lamplight when I could. That would relax him instantly. There isn't a science to this. It might be a lot of trial and error. Good thing there are twenty-four hours in a day and seven days in a week so we can learn what our babies need from us.

Also, please note: *You do not need the blessing of your twins' personal pediatrician if you'd like to seek professional help.* Most states offer free evaluations for what is typically called "early intervention." You can call your local health department for full details.

Pediatric occupational therapist Lindsey Biel, coauthor of *Raising a Sensory Smart Child*, offers the following tips for helping preemie babies with their sleep:

- Reduce overwhelming visual stimulation (an "interesting" mobile may not work for them!).
- Keep your babies swaddled for a good part of the day, but always make sure their hands are free, so they can suck on their fingers and fists when they are developmentally ready. Ensure they have opportunities each day to kick and stretch their little legs, too.
- When holding your babies, tuck in their arms and legs so that they are in a secure, flexed position, as they would be in the womb.
- Keep them warm, with a household temperature of 68 to 72 degrees and extra layers.

If your child or children are in the care of an occupational therapist (OT), make sure to speak to them about their specific recommendations.

Taking Care of You

Now that your little ones are here, you may understand why we are making a point of emphasizing self-care. Like many parents or caregivers of newborns, you are probably exhausted. And there's a lot more going on as well.

Parent Brain Development

Yes—"baby brain" is a real thing! Birth mothers temporarily lose the ability to multitask, become hyperfocused, and develop a higher sensitivity around sight and touch, according to Dr. Oscar Serrallach, an expert in the field of postnatal health and author of *The Postnatal Depletion Cure*. Their brains instinctively slow down to help them focus on their baby's subtle cues and communications.

Brain changes aren't just for birth moms, either. All caregivers exhibit them as they care for babies. When humans transition into the role of parent, major structural and functional changes occur in their brains that help them focus on caring for their infants—regardless of whether they carried and gave birth to the child. Nannies and childcare workers experience these brain changes, too (though the extent of this change depends on the amount of time they spend caring for babies). Researchers speculate that this is an evolutionary adaptive behavior that has supported the success of humans over many thousands of years. If an infant's birth mother were to die, the baby would need another caregiver or caregiver network to be able to step in.

As your twins' parent, be gentle with yourself as you find yourself becoming more sensitive and focused. For birth mothers, these changes can last up to two years. And while these brain changes can feel disconcerting, they are beneficial for helping you recognize and meet your babies' needs.

Preventing Postpartum Depletion

For birth mothers, the postnatal depletion that goes along with those brain changes is often an additional challenge. Postnatal depletion is a group of symptoms that affect all aspects of life and can stem from physiological issues, hormone changes, and the disruption of the normal circadian rhythm. While all caregivers may experience some elements of postnatal depletion—experiencing exhaustion due to sleep deprivation and feeling socially isolated as they care for their babies in the first few months—birth mothers have the additional challenge of having provided, or in the case of nursing mothers still providing, necessary nutrients to her children.

In other words, the exhaustion birth mothers feel can also be caused by the postnatal depletion their bodies may be experiencing—and, yes, a twin pregnancy will cause even more depletion.

You Need a Moment to Heal

I always try to remind all our parents who take a Twiniversity class that pregnancy and birth are rough! You need a minute to heal from it—physically *and* psychologically. I find it interesting that when I ask how my moms might help themselves heal if they broke an arm or leg, they usually say they would take time off work, take any medications prescribed by a doctor, eat nutritiously to promote healing, and get plenty of rest. But after delivering twins, they'll often put all the spotlight on their babies' well-being and none on their own. You need to be sure you're resting, eating well, drinking your water, and taking care of yourself.

Babies Blues Versus Perinatal Mood and Anxiety Disorder (PMAD)

After your twins are born, things start to get a bit wild. Odds are you'll sleep less, feel a little overwhelmed, and your life will be a blur of moments filled with poopy diapers. And while it's normal to feel different as a new mom or dad, I need you guys to be on the lookout regarding your mental health.

Odds are you've already heard of the "baby blues" (including in chapter 2 of this book!), which are typically brief episodes of mild mood changes in the first few weeks after delivery. You might find yourself having some sadness that you can't explain or even some anxiety. You may find yourself crying at television commercials or even something sweet you heard. This is all pretty typical. You're a ball of hormones that are trying to reset after delivery, and you'll have a few peaks and some valleys. It's common. But baby blues go away in about two weeks. If those feelings of intense sadness and anxiety or mood swings go on longer than that, you may be experiencing perinatal mood and anxiety disorder (PMAD), an umbrella term for a set of mood disorders that includes postpartum depression.

In birth mothers, pregnancy hormones plummet, which affects brain chemistry and contributes to what can feel like an emotional tornado. Exhaustion is a risk factor for depression. And depression makes it harder to sleep properly, which in turn breeds more exhaustion. And if you already have a history of depression, that just adds to the risk.

Traditionally, PMAD was thought to begin in the first month after birth, but now we know it can also occur later in that first year. It's not good for the parent, and it's also not good for the baby, who may have more trouble forming a secure bond with a parent who is depressed, emotionally flat, unresponsive, or anxious.

Also, note that postpartum mood disorders aren't just an issue with birth moms. This condition can also appear in fathers and adoptive parents.

If sad feelings or anxiety are overwhelming, if you experience any thoughts of harming yourself or your babies, or if your symptoms start to interfere with your daily life, please get evaluated for postpartum depression immediately. And make sure you're paying attention to your partner, too.

I had significant postpartum depression and anxiety. I personally didn't recognize it, and since I had never experienced depression before, I chalked it all up to the kind of feelings I thought any new parent would have. I was overwhelmed, to say the least. Delivering early led to a slew of guilt (I felt my body had failed me and therefore I had failed my twins) and that led to anxiety (worrying what would fail next) and then to depression, since I felt utterly hopeless that I could succeed as a mom of twins. I clearly remember saying to my sister, Vivian, a few days after I gave birth but before I was discharged, "I can't do this. We need to go. I can't be their mom." I sincerely, from the bottom of my heart, wanted to abandon my newborn twins in the NICU. I felt such shame that I delivered them at thirty-four weeks, somehow thinking it was my fault—that my early delivery was in my control. I couldn't face the doctors and nurses. I was so embarrassed. I had no idea that so many other twin moms delivered around the time I did. I had no idea it was as common as it is. It's one of the main reasons I started Twiniversity. I want folks to know what other families go through, so they never feel alone. Thank goodness for my sister, who said, "OK, let's go. Where do you want to go?" She said it so sincerely that it snapped me back into reality. Except then I felt guilty for wanting to leave them. Yeah, it was a whirlwind. Sure, not every mom or dad will go through what I did, but know that if you do, you're not alone.

I am even more thankful to my husband, John. He was the one that recognized what I was feeling as depression and helped me get the support I needed. In my book *What to Do When You're Having Two*, I call it my *Memoirs of a Geisha* moment. My husband told me that I needed to have some time to myself, and knowing how much I loved going to the movies and eating popcorn in the dark, he encouraged me to go see something I would enjoy. I went to see *Memoirs of a Geisha* because I had just finished reading the book. It couldn't tell you if I liked the movie or not, but I can tell you that it was my first moment to think about what had happened. My traumatic delivery, my anxiety, my depression . . . my loss of self-control, in many ways. From there I called my doctor, explained what was going on, and the rest, as they say, is history.

Developing PMAD does not mean you are a bad parent. It does not mean that you will not feel better or not enjoy parenthood for many years to come. It does not even mean you will experience it after every birth (although you are at higher risk). It just means your body is having a harder time regulating, and you may need some extra help. That's all. You'll be OK if you get the help you need. If you need help, ask. Or rather, don't ask—demand. Be as brutally honest as you possibly can. You need to take care of yourself, or you won't be able to take care of anyone else, especially your new-born twins.

Access Twiniversity's PMAD resources at the QR code.

Your Sleep and Well-Being

Sleep when the babies sleep? Ha!

As a new parent of twins, you get a ton of advice thrown at you left and right. Many of the wise folks giving you said advice will be singleton parents. One of the most singleton-y pieces of advice folks give is "sleep when the babies sleep." For those of you who have twins, and especially those who are breastfeeding, you'll know that it always feels like there is a baby awake. Following that line of thinking, are you supposed to do laundry when the baby does laundry? Empty the dishwasher when the baby empties the dishwasher? Uh. "Sleep when the baby sleeps" drives me nuts. We know folks mean well, but we have to be realistic. Sleep when your babies sleep is not it.

So, when *do* you sleep? Basically, you sleep when you are off duty. When is that? When your partner is on duty or when folks come over that you trust to watch the kiddos while you close your eyes for a bit.

I'd love it if you aimed for several chunks of two-hour sleep if you are breastfeeding, and a five-hour chunk, at least, if you are not, every night. While you're establishing your breastfeeding schedule with your duo, you should get up when the babies have to eat, even if you just pump and go right back to sleep. But sleeping through a feeding, while not a great idea because it could mess with your supply, isn't a deal-breaker. If you are utterly exhausted and you can't function, you need to SLEEP! We can always fix any lactation issues later. I need you to be on your game, and sleep is how that happens.

Sleep is one of the big reasons why twin families typically stay on a schedule. If your babies are on a feeding schedule, you can prepare for the help you need to put that schedule into action while also getting some rest.

 ## Twiniversity Tip

Your duo's sleep schedule is very inconsistent during this time; they will be sleeping and feeding around the clock. Plan for this by napping when you can. Heck, grab a nap when Grandma comes over, instead of staying to socialize. She will understand! Don't forget, she was a new mom, too, once.

Calming Yourself Calms Your Newborns

To help keep your kiddos regulated and calm, it's helpful to keep an eye on your own stress level. Manage it so that *you* can stay regulated (or get yourself back to a regulated state). We can do this through meditation, yoga, and/or breathing exercises. The way we respond to our twins impacts them in both the moment and the future—because it influences the development currently occurring in their brain.

I'm a HUGE advocate of meditation. If you ever met me in person, you'd think I was the LAST person who could sit quietly, but it's an amazing outlet for my stress and anxiety. Yeah, I don't mind admitting it, I have had an anxiety issue for most of my life. But it wasn't until after I had my twins that I finally sought help for it. Meditation is one of the biggest keys to my happiness. Once upon a time, I even spent months learning Transcendental Meditation (TM). I'm not suggesting that you do the same. But taking a moment for yourself, whatever form that takes, is a pretty important step that most new parents forget or dismiss.

Meditation comes in many shapes and forms. Some people sit quietly twice a day for twenty minutes while repeating a mantra in their heads (that's TM), while others listen to a guided meditation with headphones from a free video they found online. There is no wrong or right way to meditate. The whole point is to take a moment and let your mind settle. Whether you are feeling calm or like you're out of control, allow your brain to chill out at least once a day when possible. Letting your brain and body reconnect will help you think more clearly and more calmly.

Parenting twins is tough. I'm sure that's not news! And we often get caught up in the whirlwind that is our life with new babies. If you don't take a minute, you're going to miss a lot. If you can give yourself an opportunity to regroup, refresh, and reconnect with *you*, your memory will be better, you'll feel more levelheaded, and you'll be able to enjoy more parts of your day. It doesn't have to be literal meditation; it just has to be a moment when you close your eyes, catch your breath, and get ready for the next part of your day.

"What Is My Reality?"

I honestly hope when you read this you say, "Nat's nuts! Of course I'm taking great care of myself." If so, you'd be one of the few. Many new families that I've worked with over the last decade can tell me every detail about their twins' poop but are paying little or no attention to themselves.

When I meet a new family for the first time, even virtually, I'll ask the mom, "How are you doing?" She will typically reply, "We are doing good . . ." and start a mini TED Talk about what her newborn twins are up to. I'll often interrupt her and say, "No, I asked how *you* are doing. How are you eating? How are you sleeping? What are you doing to help your healing process?" Depending on how many days it's been since delivery, I'm often met with a long pause, sometimes tears, and then the truth. Sometimes moms and dads will tell me about their birth trauma, sometimes they will go into detail about how they are feeling emotionally. Sometimes they will openly cry and tell me how afraid they are.

As with so many other things, there is no right or wrong here when it comes to how you feel about all the changes you're experiencing. Everyone heals from birth differently. Sometimes there are physical scars, and sometimes there are emotional ones from a disappointing birth experience. Don't hold it in. You have to find someone you trust and let it all out to them, or it can build up and become a bigger issue in your mind. Talk to your partner about how you feel, both body and mind. Be honest. Talking to someone you trust and love is a great way to release some of your pain and anxiety. You can even give them a disclaimer before you start, like "I really need you to listen to me. I'm hurting and need to get this out."

If there is one thing you take away from this book, please let it be the parts about self-care. I wish I could cast a spell on all of you that allowed you to know what I know. That YOU matter a lot when it comes to taking care of your children. You need to take care of YOU as much as you need to take care of THEM.

Focus on the things that make you happy. If you love breastfeeding, do it as much as you like. You won't hear a negative word from me. If you hate breast-feeding, do it as little as you want. Again—you won't hear a negative word from me. Take care of YOU. Sleep. Eat well. Drink plenty of water. Rest. And most importantly, recover.

 Twiniversity Tip

It's very easy to become isolated from the world. Feel free to limit yourself to the guests you are most comfortable with. Don't feel obligated to see anyone at any time just because they want to see you. It's OK to say, "Yes, we'd love to see you. How does next Tuesday work?" Take care of yourself, please. Boundaries aren't a bad thing when it comes to you and your twinnies.

Hold Tight!

What an amazing and challenging time your twins' first month is!

I know that you are doing your best to navigate it, and you are succeeding. Sure, it may feel like you are fumbling through your days and nights, but that just means you are learning. And so are your little ones. You are doing great! And things will change before you know it. Soon your twins will be ready for more sleep shaping and longer stretches of sleep.

Don't ever feel like because you had twins you're unable to do anything. Yes, you have a bonus baby, but instead of looking at it as a half-empty glass of things you might miss, think of it as a glass overflowing with all the things you'll expe-rience. Twins are an amazing gift. I promise you that, in time, even if you are struggling today, you'll look back on this time (though it might be a little fuzzy), and you'll realize how lucky you are to have two amazing kiddos who will love you with all their little hearts.

FAST to Sleep Summary

Your babies are operating from the most primitive part of their beings. They are learning how to become humans, and that's hard work. As a new parent, you're experiencing brain changes as well that are letting you care for your duo. It's hard work, but always remember this: Many, many moms and dads have walked this path before you, and you're going to do great.

What to Focus on This Month

1. Accept help and delegate anything that isn't focusing on your healing and your newborns.
2. Learn about and avoid habituation (how babies screen out overstimulating situations).
3. Implement Kim's 3 PM Rule.
4. Focus on feeding your baby a minimum of eight times in twenty-four hours unless told otherwise by a medical professional.
5. Don't let your twinnies sleep through a daytime feeding (over three hours).
6. Help your newborn straighten out their days and nights.
7. Aim for one-to-five-minute tummy time sessions, two to three times per day.
8. Establish a daily feeding and sleep routine for both you and the twins.
9. Create a sleep-friendly environment.
10. Commit to at least one self-care activity a day . . . something just for YOU! Even if it's just listening to an episode of a podcast you love.

What Not to Worry About

Sleep training! You *cannot* create any bad habits at this age.

For a printable PDF of this month's "FAST to Sleep Summary" plus helpful book bonuses, use the QR code.

Notes

chapter four

Your Twins' Second Month

Ages 4 Weeks to 8 Weeks

> *This month, we'll share some gentle, soothing tools for both your twins*
> *and you. We'll address your twinnies' increased fussiness and look*
> *at how to soothe colic, allergies, and eczema. We'll talk about a few*
> *nighttime and nap strategies as well. (Remember to take adjusted age*
> *into consideration, especially when it comes to sleep.)*

More Predictable Rhythms and Routines

At the ripe old age of two months, your kiddos' sleeping and feeding patterns will start to become a bit more predictable. The time between feedings will start to spread out, and around six to eight weeks, you will begin to see one longer stretch of sleep during the beginning part of the night. Your babies may still be going three hours between feeds, sometimes four hours with your doctor's permission, and this will open up a whole new world for you.

As we discussed last month, routines are an important part of your babies' lives. Babies truly "live in the moment," so having a rhythm and pattern to their day gives them an inkling of what comes next. Building familiar and consistent routines around your babies' days and nights will help them feel safe and secure, and holy moly guacamole, it will help you just as much. You'll find your day falling into more predictable patterns, which will eventually help with sleep (YAY!) because it makes your twinnies easier to soothe, and the routines will cue them when sleep is "up next."

The good news is that you've probably settled into some gentle routines without even realizing it! You may sing the same song before each nap or when your babies are fussy, or perhaps you always smooch your babies' toes after a diaper change. These little acts amount to a much bigger picture for your newborns. Remember that the world is a lot to take in and can be very overwhelming to your twins' still fragile nervous systems.

Flexibility is important right now. Yes, you should still keep an eye on your feeding schedule and stay on that three- or four-hour feeding timeline, but it's also important to remember that the rest of the hours of your day should be a bit wiggly. Focus on creating a nice, consistent flow to your day. Do things in the same order on a regular basis. While doing this, observe your babies' patterns to figure out what *their* natural flow looks like and how you can blend your routines in. The early stages of twin life feel like the movie *Groundhog Day*, where you'll do the same things each day, almost at the same time, but each day you'll get a little better and master the art of twinnies a bit more.

If you are the type of person who *hates* routine, I'm sorry you feel that way, but trust me, you'll thank me later, when your twins are sleeping and eating and thriving right along with you. For routine suggestions, please see "Your Twins' First Month," page 66.

Routines Help the Village

Every now and then, I'll get a call from a family who's desperate for help. Their twins aren't sleeping, they aren't eating enough, the parents aren't sleeping, and everyone is at their wits' end. The first thing I say is, "Tell me what your day looks like. Don't skip anything. Let's start at 7 AM and run through from there."

If a family starts off by saying, "Well, some days we start our first feed at 5 AM and others we start at 6 AM, but others we start at 7 AM," I always feel like I need to pull on the proverbial reins and stop them right there. But after taking meticulous notes on their whole day, I gently tell them that, without a routine, they are feeling out of control, and therefore their babies probably are, too.

My first suggestion is to start waking their twinnies at the same time each day, change their diapers, and start their first feed. I know, I know—"never wake a sleeping baby." Yeah, skip that advice, it doesn't apply to twins. If you don't create some kind of routine, there is a good chance that you'll be feeding or shushing a baby almost twenty-four hours a day. Routines aren't bad. They help everyone.

After looking at their twinnies' wake times, we focus on feeding times, move to nap times, and cover play times, getting out of the house times, bath times, and finally bedtimes.

Once they start living their day consistently, they notice that their babies eat better, sleep better, and are generally happier—and so are they.

It's important to note that your routines don't have to be super elaborate. Before putting your twinnies down for a nap or bedtime, for example, just focus on four things that you think you can consistently do. (If I had to pick them for you, it would be feeding, dimming the lights, swaddling, and singing.) The predictability of these soothing activities will allow your twinnies to relax right along with you.

 ## Your Developing Duo

As your babies begin to reach new developmental milestones, you'll notice that there is a period of disorganization that occurs right before each burst in development. Just when you've settled into a groove or set of routines that works for your little ones (progress!), you find they're suddenly fussy at an hour when, days before, they had been consistently calm. You may think, *What the heck am I doing wrong? Are they sick? Not getting enough to eat?* Take a deep breath, this is totally normal.

Brain Development

At this point, your babies are still mostly operating from their primitive brain. They won't start using their emotional brain—which allows them to learn rudimentary ways to soothe themselves—until between four and six months. But the transition has started.

The Sensations Development

According to the well-known book on developmental milestones by Dr. Frans Plooij and Dr. Hetty van de Rijt, *The Wonder Weeks*, around week five, your babies enter a new world of sensations. At this stage, they can better see and hear their surroundings. These new senses can be exciting but also potentially overwhelming.

In conjunction with (or just before) this developmental change (or what *The Wonder Weeks* refers to as a "leap"), your twins may exhibit a fussy period, particularly demonstrating what researchers Plooij and van de Rijt call the three Cs: cranky, clingy, and crying. You can help your duo by providing the closeness they crave and helping them explore their new world—providing opportunities to use their heightened senses.

Hold on to your hats here. You're not going to want to hear this, but during this phase, crying can become excessive. Get your ear plugs ready, but more importantly, get yourself ready. To help, it's particularly important to create a calming environment in the afternoon and early evening. We will help you soothe your babies through this leap. You're gonna make it. Stay strong.

PURPLE Crying

While PURPLE crying sounds like something Prince would have written and sung about back in the day, it's a term coined by Dr. Ronald Barr, a developmental pediatrician and world expert on infant crying. (Yup, there is a world expert on crying. I think it's the first job I did not want to have.) Dr. Barr, in partnership with the National Center on Shaken Baby Syndrome (NCSBS), developed the Period of PURPLE Crying program to describe this completely normal stage of infant development, which starts around two weeks of age, peaks during the second month, and decreases by month five. The NCSBS partners with hospitals and early intervention programs to educate parents that this crying period is a normal part of development.

The PURPLE acronym highlights the identifying characteristics of this period as a reminder to parents:

P: Peak of crying

U: Unexpected

R: Resists soothing

P: Pain-like face

L: Long-lasting

E: Evening

Dr. Barr wants parents to know that although this stage can be stressful, it is a phase your little ones will move through. He wants parents to prepare for the possibility of heightened crying so that they can also learn to calm themselves as they calm their babies.

Unlike colic, it's not a diagnosis. It's just a description of what crying at this age can look like. Because we know that this age is the beginning of increased crying, this chapter will continue our focus on helping you read your twins' cues and share pointers on soothing them and you.

Supporting Development for Better Sleep

As in your twinnies' first month, there is one activity you can engage in with them that will help support their development and establish a strong foundation for self-soothing and better sleep: tummy time. Positioning them on their stomach will help them strengthen their neck and arm muscles, which will help them to roll over in the future (and let them soothe themselves by doing so, rather than having to rely on you to help them change positions).

At this age, you can work on tummy time *up to twenty or thirty minutes total per day*. Pick times when your babies are alert, aware, and social (but not right after feeding so they are less likely to spit up).

 ## Feeding

By this time, you will have started to find a good feeding pattern, and feeding itself probably has become more efficient, requiring less time. Your babies have typically regained their birth weight, and you should feel in the groove when it comes to feeding overall.

Feeding at This Age

In the second month, babies usually take between two and a half and four ounces per feeding every three to four hours, whether breastfeeding or bottle-feeding. You can expect your twins to still need feedings at night (the number of times will depend on your little one). However, they may feed fewer than eight times within twenty-four hours if they are getting more at each feeding.

The amount of milk or formula that each baby needs is dependent on their weight. So, if your twins have a significant size difference (one bigger kiddo, one tinier kiddo), they may need different amounts. It's another reminder of how critical it is that you ALWAYS remember: Your twins are just two humans born on the same day. Not everything they do will be the same. In fact, you should always assume it's NOT the same to be sure you are doing the right thing. Many times, they will be eating the same amount, but you should check with their doc to be sure. It's not as uncommon as folks think for families to have different feeding requirements for their different babies.

How Much Should My Baby Eat?

If you want to play *How Much Should My Baby Eat?*, a game show that I can't believe doesn't exist yet, remember that there is a general rule to figure this out:

Body weight (in pounds) × 2.5 = number of ounces

For example, if you have a nine-pound baby . . .

9 × 2.5 = 22.5 ounces of milk

Then, to figure out how much your baby should be getting each time they feed, divide this by the number of feeds. So, for a nine-pound baby eating eight times a day . . .

22.5/8 = *roughly* just under 3 ounces of milk per feeding

Most babies will increase the amount of breast milk or formula they drink by an average of one ounce each month before leveling off at about seven to nine ounces per feeding.

I hope you are keeping up with your sleep and feeding log. If you aren't using our Twiniversity app, which is still the only app created for twin parents by twin parents, I hope you're using a good old-fashioned piece of paper to know who is sleeping and when, and who ate what and when. Poops are important, too, and don't forget to write down any medications.

If you have been keeping a log, you may see a daily pattern emerging where there is one longer stretch of sleep between feedings at night. Your babies may then go longer between feedings in the morning and want to feed frequently toward the late afternoon and evening. Keep this new pattern in mind as you tweak their afternoon and bedtime routines.

You might be seeing something *like* the feeding times in the schedule on page 120 if your babies are eating every three hours.

For your own printable copy of this schedule, see the QR code.

Feeding Challenges in the Second Month

Addressing eating and digestion challenges continues to be one of the most important things you can do to help support sleep. It's helpful to address any outstanding feeding issues at this time with your doc, lactation consultant, or a feeding specialist you may have been referred to after your hospital discharge. But we have a few tips for the most common issues.

Latch Challenges

Breastfeeding SHOULD NOT hurt. If you have pain or discomfort for more than a few seconds, odds are, the reason is a bad latch. A proper latch is critical for breastfeeding—and not only for your comfort. Without the right placement of their lips and tongue, your kiddo will get super frustrated at not getting the nourishment they need and that will make you extremely frustrated, too.

If your twins are having issues eating, they will have issues sleeping. You, yourself, can't sleep if you're hungry, and your twins aren't any different.

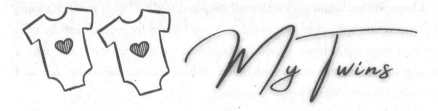

Second Month Home
Daily Schedule

Sample Schedule Based on 3hr Feedings*

6am		
7am	🩲 🍼	
8am		
9am	☕	
10am	🩲 🍼	
11am	🛒	
12pm		
1pm	🩲 🍼	
2pm		
3pm	☕	
4pm	🩲 🍼	
5pm	🛒	

6pm	🦆	
7pm	🩲 🍼	
8pm		
9pm	☕	
10pm	🩲 🍼	
11pm		
12am		
1am	🩲 🍼	
2am		
3am		
4am	🩲 🍼	
5am		

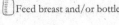 Feed breast and/or bottle    Change

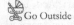 Go Outside   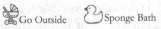 Sponge Bath   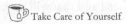 Take Care of Yourself

*Always check with your doc about schedule specifics
for your particular twins

Reflux Versus GERD

There's spit-up . . . and then there's *spit-up*!

As you learned in "Your Twins' First Month," gastroesophageal reflux disease (GERD) occurs when the valve between the esophagus and the stomach allows contents of the stomach to regularly flow back up into the esophagus and mouth. It is less common than regular spit-up, and unlike spit-up, which doesn't disrupt sleep, can seriously affect a baby's ability to rest and be happy.

If you suspect that one or both of your twinnies may have GERD, check in with your pediatrician. Much like alert babies, babies with GERD often remain sensitive to their environments even after GERD is no longer an issue. They react more to stimuli such as bright lights, crowds, food, and textures. Pay attention to their sensitivities post-GERD just as you would any baby with a sensitive temperament, and be mindful of their environment, including potentially itchy clothing and possible food triggers that might upset their tummy.

Cluster Feeding

Cluster feeding, or marathon feeding, refers to when on-demand feeding sessions bunch close together at certain times of the day and then space out at longer intervals at other times, based on a baby's particular needs and hunger cues. The bunched feeding sessions often match up with a particularly fussy time of day. In your twins' first month, you may have found yourself feeding them in multiple back-to-back sessions because they hadn't yet started settling into a feeding pattern. As a natural feeding pattern begins to emerge this month, these clusters of feeding sessions will start to stand out. Cluster feeding is normal and natural at this age, but it can feel frustrating to new parents because it may seem that their babies are fussy and eating all the time.

Cluster feeding can happen at any time of day but usually happens in the afternoon or evenings. And it's often, but not always, followed by a longer sleep period. It's as if your baby is filling their gas tank for a longer drive. Cluster feeding can be a good sign that your baby or babies are ready to sleep for longer stretches. Check with your pediatrician to confirm whether you need to wake them during this new long stretch at night to feed them.

During cluster feedings, your baby or babies may appear fussy. You may see a cycle in which they cry or pull off the breast or bottle for a minute or two and then begin to feed again. Your baby might want to remain near or on the breast or bottle for this period of time. Cluster feeding can coincide with the post–3 PM fussy period, but to be clear, they aren't just trying to self-soothe; they are pushing for more nutrition.

If you see a pattern of cluster feeding emerging, keep your schedule open during this time of day (for example, if a baby has started cluster feeding between 4 and 7 PM, don't plan to go to the grocery store).

Cluster Feeding When You Feed on a Schedule

But Nat, how will I know they want to cluster feed if I'm on a schedule? The answer is simple: If you feed them, they start to fall asleep, and they wake up cranky and start rooting, then give them a chance to feed again. Will it mess up your feeding schedule? Yes, but cluster feeding helps you produce more milk, which allows for better feeds and therefore better sleep. See, it's a chain reaction. When your twins cluster feed, they are taking more milk from you, and an empty breast really does fill up faster. They are helping you build a more significant supply. Yes, it's frustrating and time consuming, but it will be beneficial in the end.

 ## Attachment

A quick review on why attachment is important: A secure attachment is crucial to your children's future ability to interact with others, develop empathy, and self-regulate, and the key to forging a secure attachment is caregiver responsiveness. Attachment happens as you and your babies develop your own unique language and your twins learn to trust that you will help them meet their needs.

Babies learn how to self-soothe by experiencing brief moments of distress— like while learning to roll, having their diaper changed, and feeling hungry before they are fed—alongside a caregiver they trust. With your help, they experience how to go from a dysregulated state to a regulated one. Once they learn what a regulated state feels like, they learn to ask for your assistance to get there. Eventually, they learn to get there on their own through physical actions like looking away, rolling to their side, or sucking their thumb. But at this stage, they can't necessarily do these things on their own.

With the increased crying this month, you (and ALL of your babies' caregivers) will be responding more and experimenting. Remember, it's OK to get it wrong! You and your twins are still learning about each other. The important thing is just that you respond.

Consistently comforting your babies *now* lays the foundation for them to become confident and secure, and that's going to be a big help when you start sleep coaching in a few months. Don't worry about spoiling your little sweeties in these early months. Our ultimate goal is independence, and focusing on responding and being attentive now is what will get us there. I pinky promise you.

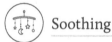 Soothing

You may have thought you were getting a handle on your duo's cues and how to soothe them, only to hit this increased fussy period and find that your best tricks no longer work, or that what works one day doesn't work the next. Continue to experiment! This section on soothing offers more ideas you can try.

As you reach the end of this month, habituation wanes, but your twins haven't yet mastered self-soothing. They are still practicing. Hey, it's a big month of learning, for them and for you! Work with what they have available to them skills-wise and keep your expectations realistic. This month it's key to be prepared to soothe post–3 PM fussiness and take advantage of your babies' developing senses in trying new calming tools.

If one or both of your twins have entered the PURPLE crying stage, they may be upset for no particular reason and simply need soothing. Developmental milestones or just an off day may cause your kiddos to fuss. That said, at this age, your babies might also be trying to communicate something to you by crying. And deciphering the meaning of their cries can be particularly important as you are trying to soothe them in preparation for sleep.

Common Causes of Crying

Feeding Issues

- Hunger (How long has it been since their last feeding? Was it a good feed? Is this a cluster feeding time of day?)
- Fast/slow milk flow (bottle or breastfeeding)
- Low milk supply or oversupply
- Possible lip or tongue tie
- Upset tummy
- Allergy

Comfort

- Diaper needs changing
- Temperature is too hot or cold
- Clothes are scratchy
- Tiredness
- Overstimulation (How long have they been awake? Babies are more easily overstimulated when overtired. Have there been any changes to their environment in the last couple of days? Are they in a loud place, like a restaurant, with siblings running around and new smells from the kitchen? Have they been handled too much by family?)

Medical

- Illness
- GERD
- Constipation
- Diaper rash
- Eczema
- Torticollis (when the neck muscles regularly contract, causing the head to twist or tilt to one side)

Keep in mind that you may not always be able to calm your babies down—you may just need to wait for the crying to pass—but being there for them, trying to help, and showing them love will make all the difference.

No one said this was going to be easy, but it will all be worth it. Twins can make you feel like you're solving a never-ending mystery, but before you know it, you'll be chief detective, able to solve any whimper and cry within seconds. It just takes practice.

Soothing Your Babies

As your twins' senses develop, they get temporarily fussier, and yet their heightened senses of touch, hearing, smell, and more will help you soothe this fussiness, including in preparation for sleep. Here we offer some ways of taking advantage of your babies' new senses. Try focusing on one sense or soothing through more than one sense at a time, if you like.

Touch

Body contact through touch activates oxytocin in the brain—which lowers the stress levels in both you *and* your babies. Touching and holding calms your kiddos and has the added benefit of bolstering attachment.

To calm your babies through touch, try:

- Rubbing their palms or clapping their hands together.
- Gently exercising their legs, waving their arms, or lifting them up and down.
- Breastfeeding (even if they have already fed, your baby will benefit from the body contact and may be soothed by non-nutritive sucking).
- Rubbing their tiny feet from toe to heel.
- Taking a warm bath or shower together. (Just MAKE SURE you have extra hands around. Babies are squirmy already; when they are slippery, keeping ahold of them is even harder.)
- Concentrating on your breathing while holding a baby close (taking a deep cleansing breath from your diaphragm and exhaling slowly and completely).

Infant Massage

When my twins were two months old, infant massage was one of the activities I most looked forward to each day in our house. Spending any relaxed one-on-one time with a baby brings only positive results for both of you, psychologically and physiologically (and for your baby, developmentally). But the benefits of stopping and really connecting with your baby through infant massage are astounding.

Infant massage has shown to help babies under six months sleep better, cry less, and feel less stressed. Massage affects their tiny bodies positively overall and can really aid in easing discomfort from gas, constipation, teething, and congestion.

Try to find some time in your schedule each day to dedicate to massage. But be flexible and watch for signs from your baby that it is time to stop: a cry, stiffening of limbs, or irritability. Your strokes should be firm and not ticklish. Research and try out some different techniques until you find the one they enjoy the most. Start when your baby is in a quiet and alert state, right after a feed or a bath, or another time when they are not sleepy.

Movement

Movement often helps to calm and settle your babies. During Twiniversity class, I demonstrate how something as simple as standing up and walking around a room can help soothe your kiddos. Think of it this way: When they were in your belly, you walked around a bit. You sat, you got up, you were in the car or on public transportation, bouncing around as you went to and from work. They were always moving right along with you. Once they're born, your movement might not lessen, but theirs does. Holding them securely and walking with a little bounce in your step, or even just walking normally, can go a long, looooooooong way toward soothing them.

You can use movement with your twin in several ways:

- Holding and rocking your babies (or swaying with your babies).
- Taking them for a walk in their stroller or carrier.
- Placing your babies in their swings or vibrating chairs (while supervised).

- Sitting on an exercise ball and bouncing with one of them. (This is also awesome for your circulation, so it's a double benefit!)
- Wearing a super fussy baby around the house in a sling or carrier, for example while putting away laundry. Just make sure that the sling/carrier is acceptable for their age and weight.
- Dancing with your baby. Recommended listening: Jennifer Lopez, Mariah Carey, Beyoncé, Ricky Martin, Celine Dion, Hillary Scott, and Chris Stapleton, just to name a few. Know why? They all have twins! They feel your struggle.

Distraction

New activities and exploring new surroundings activate dopamine, a neurotransmitter that controls the pleasure center of the brain and regulates emotional responses. When you distract your babies with new experiences, you soothe them.

You can try:

- Bringing them into a different room.
- Walking around the house or their room and pointing out various items.
- Stepping outside into the fresh air.
- Taking a walk with them in their stroller.
- Playing some upbeat music.
- Wiping their face with a wet washcloth.
- Starting bath time early.
- Pretending to sneeze (trust me, this one is silly but a doozy!)

Sounds and Smells

Sounds and smells can activate positive feelings and lower stress levels. Sometimes they can be overstimulating, though, so start slow.

In addition to white noise (see chapter 2 for more on white noise), you can try:

- Turning on the stove fan or bathroom fan.
- Turning a radio on to static.
- Playing familiar music and singing along (combine this with movement by moving both of you to the rhythm!).

- Talking quietly and soothingly.
- Playing sounds of the womb (more of a whooshing sound than white noise) or heartbeats.
- Introducing calming scents like lavender or vanilla (but do this in small doses at first so it's not too overwhelming).

When trying these soothing tools, first experiment with one at a time. If you start combining too many at once, you'll never know if only one did the trick. Also, if one tool doesn't work, take a beat before jumping to a new one. Moving between activities too abruptly could upset your baby or babies even more. Moving slowly between two soothing solutions will allow them to settle into the new activity and help you accurately test their response.

Pacifiers in Month Two

Pacifiers are particularly popular this month because they:

- Allow your baby to soothe themselves during this period of general fussiness.
- Become another soothing tool for breastfeeding mothers so that they don't have to be on call to soothe at all times.
- Can ease ear pressure during air travel—which parents may start to take advantage of more as their twinnies grow older.

As magical as pacifiers can feel, it's important to pay attention to your babies' cues so you understand when they need to feed as opposed to when they just want to soothe themselves with sucking. Remember, the pacifier is just one tool in your soothing toolbox.

Soothing Challenges in the Second Month

There are two main hurdles you may need to jump to effectively soothe your twins this month. The first is colic, which we went into in depth in "Your Twins' First

Month" on page 80. The second is overstimulation, which we introduced in the last chapter but discuss in more detail here.

Overstimulation

As your twins' senses become more developed, their brains and bodies have to start processing all of the new information that is coming their way. Overstimulation happens when they take in too much information, whether suddenly all at once or over the course of the day. All that input may become too much for their brains and/or bodies to handle. You can tell that one or both of your twins are becoming overstimulated because they tend to get fussy and are difficult to soothe to sleep.

Along with reading their cues, it helps to regularly take note of the stimulation in their environment—and not just for your babies' benefit. Overstimulation isn't just a kiddo problem; it's a parent problem, too. For both their sake and yours, you should be aware of high levels of stimulation around you and try to reduce what you can before your stimulation cup runs over and the twins, and possibly you, become fussy.

Often parents will call me worried about their twins crying for hours every evening. I'll ask if they have the TV on or who's over, trying to gauge what the stimulation level is in the house. Very often, with my prying, they figure out that there is a pattern, and often it's related to overstimulation. Parents always think that their twins will get used to the sights and sounds of their home quickly, but they don't. They don't have that skill yet. So, it's our job to do things like limit visitors and loud noises to limit stimulation overall.

 Twiniversity Tip

Sometimes it is us, the parents, who are causing the overstimulation. If you have a spouse who comes home at a particular time at night and starts playing with the twinnies right when they are trying to start winding down for the day, you may need to make a change. This can be one of the hardest things for working parents. The moment you get home, you want to snuggle those sweet babies, but the way you're engaging may be too much for them. Use that time instead to help them wind down while you wind down, too. Use your postwork time for soothing activities like reading stories and infant massage. It will be good for the whole family, not just your twins.

Habituation in Month Two

Although habituation wanes at the end of your twins' second month, as you saw in the "Brain Development" section of this chapter, they can still habituate up to that point. This makes it even more important to be aware of their environment and watch for overstimulation so that you can recognize the difference between stressful habituation and true deep restorative sleep.

You'll probably have to say no to a few family and friend invitations for the first few months of your kiddos' lives. If your twins get overstimulated easily, going to an outside event can get overwhelming real fast, and trying to soothe two kiddos at once while trying to enjoy yourself is going to be nearly impossible. I don't want to sound like a Negative Nancy here, but rather a Realistic Rita. If you want to try visiting folks and going to events, go for it—you never know how good (or bad) it will be until you try—but have your plan B ready. Know when it's time to leave, and don't feel bad about it.

If you think that one or both of your twins are habituating but aren't sure, their behavior over the next twenty-four hours will help you to know if you are correctly reading their cues: habituation leads to fussier, less rested babies.

Overstimulation Cues

Your twins are looking for you to help them when they are overstimulated. Some cues for overstimulation include:

- Intense fussiness that is difficult to calm.
- Turning their head away and sometimes back and forth like they are saying no.
- Jerkier movements.
- Clenched fists.
- Increased startle response.

- Legs pulled up on their chest.
- Avoiding eye contact.

If you use the SOAR process (page 12) to *Assess* what was happening before these cues appeared, you will likely find that some overstimulation occurred. By noting what it was for the future, you can help your little ones from heading down the path to overload again. When you see these cues, you'll want to respond quickly—before your twins move to the next stage, intense crying.

How to Hold Off a Meltdown

When I refer to a meltdown at this age, I mean uncontrollable, red-faced, and full-body crying that can be A LOT to handle and tough to soothe quickly.

If your babies have been getting hit with a bunch of stimulation ping-pong balls—radio, TV, visitors, fans, cooking smells, dog running around, siblings yelling—you can probably fend off a meltdown by simply taking them into a quiet room, turning on some soothing music, dimming the lights, and gently rocking them. If you're not comfortable holding them both at the same time, consider wearing one in a carrier and holding one in your arms. Whatever you choose to do, just do it safely, please, and peacefully. Even if you are stressed, fake it till ya make it. If you are chill, they are more likely to be chill.

You can also make plans to keep future meltdowns at bay by arranging to do any errands and outings in the morning and then staying home in the afternoon, following Kim's 3 PM Rule from page 82. You don't have to do this forever, and it will help make your evenings more peaceful and calmer. Better yet, delegate those errands to someone else!

 ## Temperament

You'll see even more of your twins' temperaments this month in the way they react to you and objects around them, including the way that they react to overstimulation. Keep in mind, however, that the increased crying toward the end of this month is not necessarily related to their temperament.

Alert Babies

What Kim calls alert babies, child temperament expert Dr. Mary Sheedy Kurcinka calls *spirited* babies (and, later on, *spirited* children). Dr. Kurcinka shares a vast amount on these babies in her fantastic book *Raising Your Spirited Baby: A Breakthrough Guide to Thriving When Your Baby Is More . . . Alert and Intense and Struggles to Sleep*. Dr. Kurcinka says these babies can appear to have additional sensory sensitivities, such as not liking large crowds, having their face washed, or wearing or being touched by certain fabrics or textures. They might not react well to a change in their schedule or environment and may also be more cautious than other babies in new environments. Their most noticeable trait, however, is their fussiness. On the fussiness scale, these babies often go from zero to one hundred in the blink of an eye.

Kurcinka writes that "20–25 percent of all babies born are spirited . . . genetically wired to be highly alert and intense." She explains that these little ones have "highly reactive arousal systems," which makes them quick to ramp up and then slow to calm down again. Kurcinka provides a helpful "zone system" for parents and other caregivers of spirited and alert babies to help identify where their baby is at the moment:

- Green zone: Everything is fine, and the baby's needs are being met.
- Yellow zone: The baby is starting to struggle and needs a response.
- Red zone: Their arousal system has been overloaded. They are distressed and in need of a massive response.

With an alert twinnie or twinnies, it's most important to catch them before they reach the red zone—particularly when you're about to start bedtime or nap time. They will be more difficult to soothe to sleep. Learning what cues they give in the yellow zone will help you know when it's time to step in with soothing.

How to Support Your Alert Baby or Babies

We've got some specific tips for caring for these little ones, who can seem completely different from those "easier" babies you've heard about:

- Feed them in a quiet room. Other babies might happily feed undistracted with the family bustling around them, but your alert baby may do better with just the two of you alone, separated from the noise.

- Respond to your alert baby quickly, because the time frame between "a smidge fussy" and "complete toxic meltdown" is shorter than with other babies. Be ready to SOAR, moving through the process quickly, and have a soothing technique at the ready for some of their common cues.

- Parents of alert babies often carry around multiple pacifiers, and sometimes a front carrier stowed in the stroller basket in case one of their little ones gets fussy and calms down when being carried.

- Set up your sleep environment carefully, as it will affect an alert baby more than the typical baby. Your alert twinnie or twinnies might be more affected by light during naps and do better with room-darkening shades, or perhaps you'll find that you need an even dimmer night-light to keep them calm during night feedings.

- Plan to be home in time for their usual afternoon nap time. Many babies will sleep on the go for up to three months (or until their circadian rhythm develops and they become more aware of their surroundings—more on these changes in future months), but your alert baby might not be so flexible about snoozing in the car or on a stroll.

- Experiment with different types of touch, like giving them a massage or trying kangaroo care. Most alert babies need extra help regulating themselves, but know that not all alert babies respond well to touch—your touch may overstimulate them further. Use trial and error here.

 ## Getting You and Your Duo to Sleep

At the beginning of this month, you are still your twins' external clock. During the next few weeks, however, their own circadian rhythms will start to emerge. You'll see them start to appear between six and eight weeks, when you'll also see that one longer stretch of night sleep we mentioned emerge—usually at the beginning of the night. The consistent and soothing routines we've encouraged you to put in place are really starting to pay off in better sleep both at night and during the day.

Wait on Sleep Coaching!

Some parents are told to start sleep training at this age and to use the "cry it out" method to teach their baby to sleep. Yeah, please don't do that. They are way too young.

The "cry it out" method is not effective for babies at this age because:

- They are still functioning from their primitive brain and therefore cannot filter out overstimulation on their own.
- They are not mentally or physically capable of soothing themselves by turning their heads away from overstimulation or sucking on their hands for comfort. They need you to soothe them. They will get there, but they aren't there yet.
- Babies have a harder time learning when they are in a dysregulated state (overly upset and crying). Having them cry in hopes they will figure it out simply won't work!

In addition, babies produce cortisol when they are stressed, and long-term exposure to cortisol undermines brain development in the parts of the brain that will help them self-soothe in the future. Unsoothed distress (for example, when a baby is allowed to cry unsupported for longer than a few minutes) is more than a baby's brain can currently handle. At this age, even a little stress can throw a baby off balance, so try to avoid it if you can.

Twin parents should wait at least four or five months before considering sleep coaching because the first several months of life are all about brain development (to make way for self-soothing) and gaining trust. Gaining trust is the building block to creating secure attachment and the development of emotional intelligence. Therefore, we focus on what we can at this stage: sleep shaping, creating supportive routines, and paying attention to feedings.

Double the Crying

While we don't recommend you intentionally let your babies cry, that doesn't mean it will never happen. If you have to allow one baby to cry or even scream for a minute or two because you need to take care of their twin, take a breath and just get to that crying baby as soon as you can. If you are caring for your twins solo, with no help at all, you'll be faced with that situation multiple times. All you can do is your best. As a twin parent, I know there will be moments that seem impossible to get through, but you will. We've all been there, and we've all had to let a twin or two cry for a few minutes while we catch our breath. It's OK. Just get to them as soon as you can. And if it gets too overwhelming, seek help from friends or family or, if you can, even paid help.

Sleep Needs in Healthy Full-Term Babies

The typical sleep average for this second month is ***ten or eleven hours at night and five or six hours during the day, spread out over several naps***—although as we learned in "Your Twins' First Month," there is a lot of variability in sleep needs in young babies. Current research has shown that there can be a variation of up to eight or nine hours in a twenty-four-hour period for babies six months and under.

Generally, newborns between zero and three months should sleep between ***fourteen and seventeen hours during each twenty-four-hour period***. This range includes both daytime naps and nighttime sleep. Most newborns can be awake for up to one hour at a time—but some for only forty-five minutes.

Night Sleep Consolidation Begins

If you have been keeping a log, you may have noticed that your babies have started to have one longer stretch of four to five hours of sleep at night (assuming your doctor said they didn't need to be woken for feedings). Yes, they will still wake frequently after this stretch—you can expect them to wake every few hours for a feeding until around their typical wake-up time for the day—but celebrate this first long period of sleep!

"Sleeping through the night" is traditionally defined as a continuous stretch of sleep between midnight and 5 AM when there is no need for parent intervention (either soothing or feeding). You'll start to see this consolidated stretch sleep appear in babies between six weeks and three months, but keep in mind that even by nine months, studies suggest that only about 50 to 80 percent of babies sleep through the night on a regular basis.

Napping

At this stage, your twinnies can only stay awake between an hour and an hour and a half before needing to sleep again. Daytime sleep rhythms are still developing (you'll hear more about this next month), but we'll give you some napping tips to get you started in the meantime.

What the Heck Is a Wake Window?

You'll hear the term *wake window* a lot in this book and in the general world of sleep, so it's worth taking a moment to explain it. A wake window is the length of time a baby can stay awake at a specific age before getting overtired and fussy and harder to get to sleep. Paying attention to wake windows can save you and your twinnies a lot of stress.

How Long Can Your Twins Be Awake?

If you're logging your twins' sleep, the following wake windows might look familiar to you:

Nap 1: one hour after waking for the day.

Nap 2: ninety minutes after waking from nap 1 (if nap is longer than forty-five minutes).

Nap 3: about ninety minutes after waking from nap 2 (if nap is longer than forty-five minutes).

Nap 4: about ninety minutes after waking from nap 3 (if nap is longer than forty-five minutes).

Evening bedtime: about one hour after waking from a short nap 4 (under forty-five minutes) or ninety minutes after waking from a longer nap 4.

As you can tell from this list, when naps are shorter, your kiddos' awake time will also be shorter. If your baby or babies sleep for forty-five minutes or more, they will likely be able to stay awake for an hour and a half. If they sleep for less than forty-five minutes, they may only be able to stay awake for forty-five minutes to one hour.

Many babies are awake for a shorter amount of time in the morning, after which the time between naps remains fairly consistent for the rest of the day. The trick is to watch for tired signs while paying attention to how long your babies can naturally stay awake at this age—and then try to put them down to sleep before they become overtired.

Supporting Your Babies' Sleep

You're starting to see a longer stretch at night, your twins have a consistent start to their day, and you've implemented a regular bedtime routine, but are there other things you can do to support the lengthening of their nighttime sleep? Yes!

We encourage you to focus on looking for and then supporting your babies' longer stretch at night. The best way to do this is to work with where your twinnies are developmentally by following the Baby-Led Sleep Shaping guidelines below.

The Elements of Baby-Led Sleep Shaping (Month Two)

1. Create a sleep-friendly environment for your duo, which should include:
   - Room-darkening shades.
   - Soothing colors.
   - White noise.
   - Cool temperature.
2. Create daily routines:
   - At bedtime, use a consistent, soothing routine. Do this in your twins' nursery if you plan to eventually transition them there, even if you are currently room sharing.
   - Create a shorter pre-nap version of your pre-bed routine.

3. Prevent overstimulation by following Kim's 3 PM Rule.

4. Don't let your twins sleep through daytime feedings (i.e., over three hours at a time).

5. Have each twin's last nap end one hour to ninety minutes before their bedtime.

6. Support your twins' budding circadian rhythms:
    - Watch their wake windows.
    - Dim lights at night.
    - Expose them to sunshine in the morning.

7. Regulate your twins' wake-up. For example, always wake them for the day at 7:30 AM.

8. Regulate your twins' bedtime. Note the time that they usually fall asleep for the night and set that time as their bedtime.

9. Focus on creating one longer stretch of sleep at night. Try a dream feed to see if it helps (see below).

10. Fill your twins' daytime sleep tanks:
    - Help them get naps any way you can: rocking, holding, pushing them in the stroller.
    - Watch for their sleepy cues and avoid letting them get overtired.

Incorporate a Dream Feed

You might experiment with *dream feeding* at this stage. Your twins' developing circadian rhythms typically drive the deepest and longest stretch of sleep at the beginning of the night, starting at bedtime. The goal of a dream feed is to push this long stretch to their second sleep stretch of the night by regulating their first feeding, which allows you to get a good stretch of sleep, too.

Dream feeds can also be helpful during growth spurts—it lets your babies get the extra calories they need without an extra waking at night due to hunger. If you're waking them to eat on your terms, the feed is easier to manage and you avoid the stress of crying twinnies.

How to Dream Feed in Five Steps

1. Wake ONE baby between 10 PM and midnight, before you go to bed.
2. Quietly change their diaper.
3. Nurse or bottle-feed them.
4. Put them right back down to sleep.
5. Repeat with the other baby.

(Note: If your doc has recommended that one or both of your twinnies need to be held upright after each feeding, please make sure you never skip that step.)

It's also worth noting that dream feeds only work for 50 percent of babies. If, after three days, you find that doing the dream feed just adds another waking and feeding, stop and allow your twins to take their longest stretch at the beginning of the night.

Fill Your Twinnies' Daytime Sleep Tanks

Believe it or not, when babies sleep well during the day, they are more likely to sleep better at night. As you've seen, I often compare a baby's tummy to a gas tank. Well, your twinnies also have a sleep tank, and it's important to keep that full any way you can. This means, at this stage, go ahead and rock them to sleep, allow them to fall asleep at your breast, use a pacifier, or let them sleep in your arms—whatever, just get them to sleep for as many naps as you can during the day.

Is There Such a Thing as Too Much Daytime Sleep?

It is true that, for some babies, getting too much daytime sleep can result in a loss of sleep at night. If your babies' naps are so long that they do not eat regularly enough to get the calories they need during the day, they are more likely to wake up hungry at night.

If your babies are napping so long during the day that they are sleeping through feedings and it seems to be negatively affecting their nighttime sleep, it may be a result of day/night confusion. Make sure that they get enough stimulation, light, activity, and fresh air during the day. You can review our tips for resolving day/night confusion on page 92.

Avoid Overtiredness

The most important thing to keep in mind about daytime sleep is that we don't want your babies staying awake too long and getting overtired. This not only affects their mood (and yours) but also impacts their sleep quality and length during the day and at night. It makes it more difficult for them to fall asleep for the next sleep period and causes fragmented sleep cycles, resulting in shorter or restless naps.

To prevent overtiredness, make sure to watch for their sleep cues. See page 96 for a list of what to look for. The only addition this month is that they might now be able to look away from you—perhaps to stare at a wall—if they feel overtired.

Since daytime sleep is still not organized (that is, naps are still at irregular times and are irregular lengths, making your day feel a bit all over the place), your babies may be taking several long naps, or they may still be taking a number of shorter naps. If your twins consistently take short naps, you will find that they may need more naps in the day to avoid being overtired at the end of the day—often as many as four to seven. Yes, I'm serious. I know it seems like a lot.

If your babies are sleeping for longer periods of time, you will likely still find that they need three to four naps a day until they are closer to six months old.

 Twiniversity Tip

Understand that there is NO predictability in your babies' naps at this age. Take each nap as it comes and don't worry. There's a lot of growing and changing ahead!

Here is what you can focus on to support your duo's nap quality and length:

- Keep the environment calm to see if overstimulation has been causing shorter naps.
- Experiment with putting your babies in a cool, quiet, dim place for naps to see if that helps them sleep longer.
- Some babies sleep better while in the same room with a parent. You can try keeping them close by in a twin bassinet.

- Some babies sleep better in motion. At nap time, you can try taking them for a long walk in a carrier or stroller.
- If their previous nap is short, make sure you keep their next wake windows short, too—just an hour—since a shorter nap means they can't stay awake longer without getting overtired.
- Sometimes you can lengthen a nap by:
  - Soothing your baby or babies back to sleep by shushing them, patting them, or even picking them up and feeding them.
  - Watching the clock. If one or both of your babies wake consistently after twenty or thirty minutes, try setting an alarm so you can go in just before their predicted wake time and try to encourage them to fall back to sleep before they're fully awake. This will be easier than waiting until they have woken up all the way.

If either of these approaches are not working after five to ten minutes, or your baby is crying, simply end the nap and try again next time.

Babies under three months often thrive quite nicely on short power naps; it is their parents who have a more challenging time with it. If your baby has reflux, short naps can be common and may not lengthen until the reflux is under control or your baby is older—so you can hold off on lengthening strategies at this time.

 Twiniversity Tip

If you usually hold your babies until they fall asleep and you want to put your baby down, but find they that they wake the minute you do, try these tips:

- Hold them for at least fifteen minutes after they first fall asleep, until they are sleeping more deeply, before putting them down.
- Once you put them down, stay by their side. If they jolt awake, pat and shush them back to sleep. You can try this for a period that feels comfortable; many families try for about ten minutes before assuming the nap is over.

Room Sharing This Month

It's helpful to re-evaluate how room sharing is working for you and your family each month. You may need to push your twins' bassinets or cribs a bit farther away from the side of your bed to prevent sleep disruption. As you learned in the development section, their various senses are becoming stronger, which means they are more likely to hear you when you go to bed at night or see you if they wake slightly and open their eyes.

Going Off Duty

During the second month of your twins' lives, we typically ask families if they can start dividing and conquering. Is it possible for you and your partner to split the night up into shifts and take turns resting? If you think you're ready to brave a shift alone, here are some tips for making your off-duty shifts more restful.

- Really go off duty. Close your door and leave the world out there while you focus on yourself for a bit.
- Make sure your babies are with someone you trust.
- Make your bedroom your sanctuary. While you're getting some well-deserved rest, have the babies sleep in a different room.
- Close the shades or buy yourself a face mask to block out light. Bonus points if you get a sleep mask that also has Bluetooth speakers to play some relaxing music to block out any sounds.
- If you need to charge your phone, move it away from your bed to an area where you'll have to stand up to look at it. If you keep it close by, you might be tempted to keep checking it.
- Be respectful of your partner's time when *they* are off duty. Kindness, consideration, and tenderness go a long way in keeping your partnership strong.

If you are breastfeeding and are off duty during a feed, ask your partner to bring in your pump twenty minutes before your babies are due to eat, along with a snack and a glass of water. You can pump for those twenty minutes, your partner can pick it up, and you can go right back to sleep. Try to empty your breasts as much as you can so you don't become engorged and uncomfortable.

The On-Duty Parent

You got this! Being the one on duty can be a bit stressful at first, but you'll get the hang of it—and never forget that help, if you absolutely need it, is just a closed door away. When you're on duty, try to have everything at hand you need, especially if it's from the room where the off-duty parent is. If you are bottle-feeding, have your bottles ready to go, and keep a stash of clean diapers at your fingertips.

Try not to stress too much as the on-duty parent. Hopefully, you're being respectful of each other's rest and are using the time you have off duty to fill your own sleep tanks.

Back to Work

Many parents plan to head back to work sometime during this month. For back-to-work resources, including a child-care checklist and tips on breastfeeding for working mothers, please see the QR code.

Ready for More Sleep Shaping?

Toward the end of this month, if you feel you have easier babies—meaning their cues are clear and they fall asleep quickly without much fuss—you can skip ahead to next month's "Sleep" section and try practicing the Jiggle and Soothe method as a Baby-Led Sleep Shaping technique that is a nice way to prepare them for Sleep Coaching. Remember, you can always try and then decide to stop if you feel that your baby isn't ready.

Taking Care of You

Please do not skip over this section!

Ten Minutes a Day

Yes, your twinnies are still not sleeping a lot, but you've gotten through the first month and are starting to put routines in place. That makes this a great time for putting a schedule in place for yourself as well.

Do you think you can find ten minutes each day to focus on yourself? Can you help make sure your partner has ten minutes, too? You can spend those minutes in whatever way you choose. Meditating, in the shower, walking around the block with the dog—whatever you choose, just make sure it happens.

Trust me here, you NEED to take ten minutes a day for yourself. If you can grab more, go for it, but I know two hours to go to the gym or four hours to play a round of golf isn't realistic when your twins are two months old. You'll get there, I promise, but for now, you are still healing and your babies need you nearby.

Be gentle with yourself and your partner. Please.

Don't Fall for the Smoke and Mirrors

Social media and television often make parenting seem like a dream come true. You see images of new moms holding their new babies in their perfect homes with their hair done perfectly with the caption "This is what love looks like." I'm not saying that new moms don't love their babies. I'm just saying that they're posting only the picture-perfect moments and not necessarily the truth.

It's worth remembering that influencers are really just models. They get paid to look good. And many times, they're there either because they're paid to be there or because the algorithm, which is designed to keep you using social media as long as possible, knows they'll keep you shame scrolling for longer.

When these visions of social media parenting perfection pop up, they might make you feel less than. Please don't. Know you are amazing and perfect just the way you are. You made FREAKING LIFE! You're outstanding, and I'm proud of you.

Just Because You Can Do Something Doesn't Mean You Should

Social media is a very touchy subject to me because often when I'm working with new families, I have to help them unlearn things they saw while scrolling. They try tips and tricks they have seen from unvetted folks online, and some of those tricks aren't great. Kim and I believe in evidence-based and time-tested methods, like the ones you'll read about in this book and on Twiniversity.com and Kim's website, SleepLady.com—online sources where you'll find information and tips you can trust.

Avoid Gatekeeping

Repeat after me: "Yes, thank you." This should be your new mantra when folks offer to help. Caring for twinnies is a team sport, and by *team* I mean a football team and not just a team of two. If folks offer to help, even with small things, and you're comfortable with it, take the assist!

While the parent who spends the most time with the twins will have the most experience reading their cues, it is important to trust that the kiddos will be well cared for by the other parent and other trusted adults, too. Gatekeeping often starts with the primary caregiver's feelings but can be affirmed by partners and grandparents who fear that they will not care for the twins in the way that the primary caregiver wishes. It's important for everyone involved to work together to prevent this perception.

Looking back on my early parenting years, I was the QUEEN of gatekeeping. I had my family on such a tight leash that they didn't have any flexibility to learn things on their own. This went for my husband, too. Honestly, it's one of my biggest regrets, because I limited my family's learning and painted myself into a corner, so to speak. I WAS the only one who could help my twins because I never allowed anyone else to "learn" them. This was a baaaaaaad move on my part.

You can avoid gatekeeping by:

- Trusting your partner. If you aren't confident that their skills are up to the level needed to take care of your duo, consider taking a class together.
- Writing out your daily routines. That way, others can benefit from what you know when you're out and about or resting.

- Splitting things fifty-fifty from the start. Instead of taking on all the responsibilities all the time, have a conversation PREDELIVERY, if possible, about how you can divide things up.
- Not judging. If you judge the way others care for your kids, they might feel incapable of doing the right thing by you.
- Creating a chore chart, like the one we have at Twiniversity, to give all your extra hands a chance to *choose* how to help you. Not everyone who wants to help wants to help with the babies. If you have a list of items that need to be taken care of, add them to the chart and have your helpers pick what they want to do.

You need a break. And if you gatekeep too much, folks will stop asking if you need help, and NO ONE wants that. You really do need a team here to help you avoid burnout.

Congratulations!

You've learned a lot about your twins over the last two months, especially about how to soothe them. Please remember that even if you don't succeed in deciphering their cues the first time, (a) you are responding to them, which is the MOST important part, and (b) you are getting more practice, which helps you get better at it.

FAST to Sleep Summary

This month it's all about finding your groove and figuring out the best way to soothe your tiny beasts. Maybe you're just getting home from the NICU or maybe you've been home this whole time, but life is starting to settle in a bit and you are gaining insight on what makes your Baby A and Baby B tick. You are doing an amazing job, and yeah, it's not easy, but you'll get the hang of it. Twins are an absolutely amazing gift and well worth all the challenges.

What to Focus on This Month

1. Aim for up to twenty or thirty minutes of tummy time, two to three times per day.

2. Consider keeping a feeding and sleep log (I recommend our Twiniversity app) to look for emerging daily patterns, including that one longer stretch of sleep between feedings at night. Your twins may then go longer between feedings in the morning and cluster feed toward the late afternoon or evening.

3. Remember that your twins are in the PURPLE crying period and that this increased fussiness is normal because of natural developmental changes, and it will lessen next month.

4. Experiment with our list of soothing tools. Remember to try one at a time so you know what is and isn't working.

5. Put in place the Baby-Led Sleep Shaping elements (page 137).

6. Try out dream feeds.

7. Commit to taking ten minutes a day for yourself.

What Not to Worry About

Nap lengths and sleep training in general. Remember, you are NOT creating bad habits! Especially at this age, there's no wrong way to get your babies the sleep they need.

For a printable PDF of this month's "FAST to Sleep Summary" plus helpful book bonuses, use the QR code.

Notes

chapter five

Your Twins' Third Month

Ages 8 Weeks to 12 Weeks

This month we will cover sleep changes and other developmental milestones you might be seeing at this age. We'll look at growth spurts, teething, feeding strikes, and food sensitivities. We'll also talk about more calming and soothing strategies, and how to support your duo's emerging sleep schedule. (Remember to take adjusted age into consideration, especially when it comes to sleep.)

The Emergence of a Schedule

Sound the trumpets! (Insert trumpet sounds.) If you haven't already, you'll start to notice your twinnies sleeping for longer stretches during the first part of the night. This is because your babies are starting to produce and secrete their own melatonin, the hormone we release when our environment becomes dark. Melatonin helps set our internal clock (our circadian rhythm) by making us feel drowsy. It tells us when to be asleep and when to be awake. This internal clock is supported by a consistent schedule of going to bed and waking up at approximately the same time each day.

You can support your twinnies' emerging circadian rhythms in the evening by dimming the lights and creating a quiet environment that sets the stage for a soothing bedtime routine. If you keep your babies up past their natural bedtime and expose them to more light, they stop secreting melatonin and appear to get a second wind. It's the same as if you tried to fall asleep after downing a double espresso. Your little ones will be even more difficult to get to sleep for the night. So, try not to miss that window if you can.

You can actually make light work for you as well. To help your twins (and you) stop secreting melatonin during the day, try opening the shades wide in the morning, turning on all the lights, and going out for a walk in the daylight.

As your kiddos' internal clocks develop, you will start to develop a schedule, too. You may notice that your newborns start to wake more consistently around 7 or 7:30 AM and are ready for a nap again around 9 AM. If you are having trouble seeing a schedule this month, we will help you figure out where to look and how to encourage and further it. Having a feeding and sleep rhythm helps bring predictability to your day, which often means a sense of calm for you and your babies.

Returning to Work

If you're planning on going back to work this month, this new predictability makes it easier. You'll be able to tell your twinnies' care provider roughly what to expect throughout the day—when your babies tend to nap and how often they eat. It makes it easier to make appointments with your pediatrician and plan walks outside, too.

But it can also make it harder to go back to work, since things are getting easier and even a little fun. Your twinnies are starting to become little people and showing their sweet little personalities, too. The combination of this more reliable schedule, your parenting confidence, and a bit of FOMO (fear of missing out) might make heading back to the office feel bittersweet.

Your Developing Duo

Your babies' brains and bodies continue to develop and change. Most of these changes will appear at the end of the month, but there are a *few* you might notice right away.

Say Cheese

One of the all-time best parenting/baby milestones is that big gummy smile! This month, you'll notice that you are getting noticed. Your twinnies have learned to smile, and they are working it! Enjoy every second—this is one of the first (of many) rewards you'll receive from your duo.

Vision, Taste, and Smell

By two months of age, babies have developed about 90 percent of their vision and are able to focus on objects about eight to twelve inches from them—about the length of their arm. They can detect light and dark but can't see all of the colors yet.

Their improved eyesight means they can start to track you and their twin. So, if you are walking around the house and you feel like someone is watching you, you're right . . . it's one or both of your twins.

Their ability to track you and the items around them can affect your twinnies' sleep, as they may become more aware of when you are in their sleep space. But they are also more aware that their twinnie is in their sleep space, which can be a major comfort to them.

Babies can also smell their parents. No matter if you are breastfeeding or not, when you are nearby, they know. Although taste and smell develop in utero, they get even better at this age.

These changes in awareness, and the upcoming changes in their sleep cycles that cause a "mini awakening" every 45 to 120 minutes, can together mean that these mini wake-ups between sleep cycles turn into full-blown wake-ups if your babies sense you in their sleep space. You might need to move their cribs farther from your bed if you are room sharing.

At this stage, your twins might also have a more difficult time falling asleep in a brightly lit room, so room-darkening shades can be very helpful. This applies to both naps and night sleep.

It's Here! Their First Step to Self-Soothing

By three months of age, infants can intentionally bring their hands in front of their face (often called their midline). This means they can start to get their fingers, thumb, and even their fist into their tiny mouths. Once their hands can move in front of their face, they are closer to being able to soothe themselves by sucking on their fingers or thumb.

Supporting Development for Better Sleep

According to *The Wonder Weeks*, at the end of this month, your babies will begin to enter the world of "smooth transitions." Their actions will become more fluid as they gain control over more aspects of their bodies. At this age, many babies will be able to turn their heads in a fluid motion that allows them to turn away from overstimulation and keep themselves from getting overly fussy before sleep. They may also be able to roll from their tummy to their back with assistance, which means that they are on their way to rolling over on their own (some babies may already be there this month).

As a reminder, it's pretty standard for babies to be fussy and clingy before they go through a set of developmental changes. Just know that the new skills they are learning will make it worth it!

Tummy Time

At this stage, your babies will start to roll with assistance. Tummy time is the best way to help them develop the muscles they'll need in their backs, arms, and shoulders to start rolling on their own.

You can work on tummy time for **_up to forty-five or sixty minutes a day, broken into sessions_**—with the permission of their doctor. Because your twins might have been born on the earlier side, make sure you are checking in with their doc every month about expanding any time between feedings, increase in tummy time, and anything else that may be on your mind.

You'll start realizing how lucky you are to have twins during tummy time. Your twinnies will always try to find each other in addition to you, and you can use this to your advantage when it comes to tummy time. Try placing them both on the floor, head-to-head, and watch how they will try to look at each other. If you place them next to each other, be sure to change up which twin is on which side so they aren't only looking one direction.

When deciding when to have some tummy time, pick times when your babies are alert, aware, and social (but not right after feeding so they are less likely to spit up).

 ## Twiniversity Tip

Avoid container baby syndrome, which is when parents rely on devices to hold their twins so often that it doesn't allow them to develop the proper muscles. Keeping them on their back in a pack and play, their bouncy chairs, swings, or any "container" can really hurt their physical development. Pay attention to tummy time as much as you do to feedings and sleep. It really is just as important and often overlooked.

 ## Feeding

As your babies' circadian rhythms are developing, you may now begin to experience at least one longer, more consolidated stretch of sleep between feedings at night. This stretch can be between four and six hours at the beginning of the month and might even be between six and eight hours at the end of the month. This change to your twinnies' sleep means a change to their eating patterns, too!

Feeding at This Age

On average, babies in month three typically feed ***every three hours during the day*** and may go one longer stretch (between four and six hours) without eating at night. Breastfed babies may still be getting eight feedings every twenty-four hours, while bottle-fed babies might have dropped one feeding at this point.

Pay attention to how your twinnies' feedings affect their sleep. Are they feeding for a longer period of time before they sleep a longer stretch? Are they "snack feeding" in addition to their regular feeds for comfort? Try to take a look at their cues and remember there are other ways to soothe your twinnies besides feeding.

 Twiniversity Tip

Remember, if your doctor says that your babies still need to feed overnight, you have to take that advice. There are a lot of factors that come into play, including weight, gestational age, and more, and we can't determine them for ourselves. Your pediatrician will guide you in the right direction, so please make sure you're listening to them 100 percent of the time.

Your twinnies are going to take that long extended stretch without feeding only once in each twenty-four-hour period, so regular feedings every three (or four hours) during the day will help to ensure this long stretch comes at night. That may mean waking them for feeding time during the day if it approaches and they are still napping. Remember, sometimes you do want to wake a sleeping baby—or babies, in our case.

Your babies will typically experience a major growth spurt at the end of this month, so you may notice feeding patterns shifting again around their eleventh week. You may also see some broken sleep or wakings. This is normal and natural, so try not to worry. This disruption might last for a few days (both day and night) before it evens out again.

If your babies are eating every three hours during the day, their schedule may look similar to the following—especially if you are pushing the time between feeds a little longer overnight (with your doc's permission, of course).

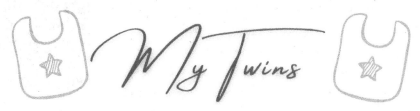

Third Month Home
Daily Schedule

Sample Schedule Based on 3hr Feedings*

6am		6pm 🦆
7am 🩲🍼		7pm 🩲🍼
8am		8pm
9am ☕		9pm ☕
10am 🩲🍼		10pm 🩲🍼
11am 🚼		11pm
12pm		12am
1pm 🩲🍼		1am 🩲🍼
2pm		2am
3pm ☕		3am
4pm 🩲🍼		4am 🩲🍼
5pm 🚼		5am

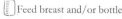Feed breast and/or bottle Change

Go Outside 🦆Sponge Bath ☕ Take Care of Yourself

*Always check with your doc about schedule specifics
for your particular twins

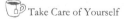

For your own printable copy of this schedule, use the QR code.

If your baby has already shifted to feeding every four hours and your doctor has signed off on this, you can see page 186 in the next chapter for what a typical four-hour feeding schedule might look like.

Supporting Sleep Through Feeding

If you aren't yet seeing one longer stretch of sleep at night, you might want to consider adding a dream feed (more in "Your Twins' Second Month," page 138). Dream feeds are one of my secret weapons for new families. A dream feed gives you the chance to fill up your babies' bellies again right before you go to bed, which encourages a longer stretch of sleep after. If you skip a dream feed, you may find yourself waking to a hungry baby or two only minutes after your head hit hits that pillow. Getting ahead of their hunger is a win-win. They get a nice full belly, and you get some extra rest!

Feedings at Night and Heading Back to Work

Depending on how your babies are sleeping at night, and if their doctor-recommended feeding schedule allows it, they may wake to eat only once a night toward the end of this month. In some rare cases, they may actually sleep through the night. If, instead, you find yourself still waking more than a few times, stay steady! Your rest will come—it just may not be time yet for your particular babies.

If you are heading back to work, you may decide to keep one or more night feedings in the schedule so you aren't making too many changes at once. You may also consider doing this to make sure that they are getting enough nutrition and to keep your milk supply consistent if you are breastfeeding or pumping. This night feed can be a really sweet time to connect with your kiddos after being separated during the day. It's OK to keep this feeding even if your twins don't need it. Please do what you need to do to make the adjustment for you and them as smooth as possible.

Feeding Challenges in the Third Month

Put fixing any feeding issues at the top of your priority list. We want to make sure that when your duo is developmentally ready for more sleep shaping and, later, sleep coaching, that a feeding challenge or two is not holding you all back.

If you aren't already, start logging your twins' feedings (time and amount) and sleep (time and length) so you can quickly start solving any problems. You can combine this information with your twins' growth curves, tracked by your doctor, to help you know if there are any issues worth discussing.

Distracted Feedings

Because your twinnies are more aware of the sights and sounds around them, it may cause some feeding distraction. Your kiddos are getting a little FOMO when eating because they just figured out that life is awesome, and they don't want to miss a thing. Think about it, would you want to stop to have a meal if you had just discovered a magic land filled with puppies and rainbows? They're just figuring out what puppies and rainbows are. Eating is boring in comparison!

To help keep your twinnies focused, consider moving to a quiet room in your home with as little distraction as possible. Note I said "as possible." If you have older kids, you can't just escape somewhere calm since you'll have to keep an eye on them, too. Think about how you might be able to limit distractions while feeding, and if you can't limit them all, what you can limit. Can you put the dog in a different room? Can you dim the lights? Can you shut a window so there is no breeze coming in? What changes can be made easily? Make 'em if you can.

Got (Less) Milk?

As your babies start sleeping for longer stretches, consider how that might affect your milk supply if you're breastfeeding. Make sure you are pumping or nursing consistently. If you are nursing and/or pumping less, you may be producing less. While technically your milk supply should follow the age and weight of your babies, when you have a duo, Mother Nature has to work twice as hard to make sure you have enough. The second month is also typically when moms of twins throw in the towel on breastfeeding. It can be tough. Trust me, I know. But if you have a particular goal in mind for how long you want to breastfeed or a date you want to hit, stay consistent with your pumping and/or nursing. You can even add a power pumping session or two per week to see if that helps you increase your supply. When in doubt, call your local lactation guru, and they can help you work out a schedule.

Nursing Strikes and Bottle Refusal

Some parents find, this month, that their babies go on a feeding strike—either refusing to nurse or refusing the bottle. It's more common than you'd think.

Feeding strikes disrupt sleep because a baby who is not getting enough nutrition during the day might turn to cluster feeding early in the night or even throughout the night. They might move to a *reverse cycle* where they are feeding more at night than during the day (see the following section).

Some parents experience feeding strikes when they first introduce a bottle to their breastfed babies. If you are seeing a feeding strike related to this, examine your bottle. Is the flow too fast? Too slow? Is the nipple too short? Too long? Your twins could be experiencing a Goldilocks moment where they are trying to find the one that is jussssst right.

If you are just introducing bottles this month, consider starting with paced feeding. Have you heard of paced feeding yet? Well, if you haven't, no worries. I'll fill you in. Paced feeding is a feeding technique that allows your babies to have a bit more control during their meals. Instead of popping a bottle in their tiny mouths and letting them gobble up every drop, you allow them to take breaths between sips and look for cues that they are asking for more. You might notice their little tongues touching their lips, signaling they are still hungry, or them blatantly opening their mouths asking for more. Or, thanks to the slower pace, you might even notice them spitting milk out, sending you the signal that they've had enough. Paced feeding is something that has traditionally been done with premature babies but is becoming much more mainstream and often recommended for full-term babies, too.

When doing paced feeding, start off with a good level 1 nipple, one of the slowest-flowing nipples, and go slow and steady. There's no rush. Bottle-feeding isn't a Nathan's Hot Dog Eating Contest. Let your babies have a chill and relaxing meal from their bottles. See how that goes and modify from there. If you see that they are getting frustrated because they aren't getting enough, quicken your pace. If you see that they aren't swallowing what's in their mouth and are overwhelmed, slow your pace. There is no right or wrong here. Just be consistent.

Don't be surprised if you notice that each of your babies has a different pace. It happens often. That's why you should always remember they are two separate people with the same birthday.

If you find yourself dealing with a nursing strike, we recommend seeing a trusted lactation consultant for help.

Reverse Cycling

Reverse cycling happens when your twin or twins start associating nighttime with eating. Typically, this occurs when your kiddo or kiddos aren't getting enough to eat during the day, either because they are distracted or on a feeding strike.

If you find one or both twins eating often at night, it's worth checking first whether they are able to go two and a half hours or longer without feeding (this might be easier to test during the day). If they aren't—if they tell you that they are ready to eat in less than two and a half hours—first check your milk supply or formula amounts and work with your pediatrician or a lactation consultant to make sure that they are getting enough to eat during the day. That may solve the problem. If they are able to go three hours without asking to be fed, hunger may not be the issue—something else may be going on. If you see this happening, don't worry, but make sure you bring it up to your doctor. It could be something small like reflux making your baby or babies not want to eat, but something a bit more serious could be going on in their itty-bitty GI tract.

To make sure that your twinnies are getting enough to eat during the day, so that they're not waking more than necessary at night, try the following:

- Feed in a place that is not stimulating: low lights, quiet, no television, no cell phone, etc.
- Ensure that they eat something every three to four hours, even if they won't take or don't seem to need a full feeding.

- If nursing, consider offering more frequent nursing sessions during the day.
- If bottle-feeding, offer more ounces in each daytime bottle to see if they will take them in.
- Don't let your babies sleep or drift off midfeeding.

 ## Attachment

Attachment, as you know by now, is built up over time. It isn't something that is there one day, gone the next, and then perhaps back the day after that. Even if you have an off day where you don't feel that you and your twinnies bonded, or where you didn't correctly interpret their needs the first time, the attachment that you've built so far doesn't just disappear.

It's important that you also remember that creating a strong attachment doesn't mean your twins don't ever get stressed. It just means that you have their backs, and you're always there to help them out. Also, just because they have called out for you does not mean you need to go to them immediately. You can let them know with your voice that you'll be on your way to them. This interaction lets them know that you've heard them and builds their trust in you. This trust helps solidify their sense of safety, which in turn helps them sleep better during naps and at night.

Consistent schedules are also key to building trust because they let your kiddos know what to expect next. For example, they might learn that after their morning wake-up, you open their curtains and sing them a good happy song before you change their diapers and put them in clothes for the day. Your babies begin to trust they will experience this series of events day after day.

You can take advantage of your twins' emerging schedule to double down on your commitment to routines throughout the day and evening. You'll have mini routines that you engage in before feedings and walks, during and after tummy time, and more. Keep repeating the routines that work and adjust those that leave one or both of them feeling a bit fussy. We want routines to be everyone's friend.

If your babies are sleeping in their own room, the pre-night sleep routine is particularly important. It is a chance for you to solidify your mutual attachment before you separate for a longer period of time.

Soothing

As you learn to read your babies' cues and respond appropriately, you are bonding, and your twins are learning to trust you. And you are learning to trust yourself as an expert on your twins! As you reflect on which soothing and calming strategies have and haven't been working for you and your duo, you will continue to add strategies to your soothing toolbox—and your babies will add their first self-soothing tool to a soothing toolbox of their own!

Self-Soothing Through Sucking

You should see that your twinnies have started sucking on their own hands. How cute! Before they get to their thumb or fingers, most babies begin by sucking their wrist and then the back of their fists. (You can trim or file their nails so that they don't accidentally scratch themselves with those tiny claws.)

By six weeks, your twins will occasionally have been able to get their hand into their mouth for a short period of time. At eight weeks, they are even better at this, and their fists begin to unfurl. They may gradually experiment with sucking on different fingers or a thumb.

If you notice one or both of your twinnies sucking on their fists and you think they may be using sucking to soothe themselves, take note of their environment. Is the room loud? Is someone in their face? Are they are getting tired? Their sucking can be a clue that will help you learn what stresses them out.

Soothing Challenges in the Third Month

At the end of the third month, colic starts to resolve. If you're finding that the crying and fussy symptoms of colic are not dissipating, your twinnies may have GERD or allergies. Make sure you're aware of the signs of GERD and check with your pediatrician for an official diagnosis. And please check out our suggestions for alleviating GERD in Months One and Two (pages 61 and 121).

If your babies suffer from eczema—dry, itchy patches on the skin—their sleep can suffer due to discomfort. Grab a tip out of the "strange enough that it just might work" jar and use some of your own breast milk on a cotton ball to treat their eczema. Because of all the amazing infection-fighting antibodies in your breast milk, it can actually help your babies' skin. Of course, if they are struggling, make sure you speak to your doc. There are a lot of different things you can try to help those sweet little babies.

 ## Temperament

As more of your kiddos' temperaments emerge this month, you'll be able to incorporate this new understanding of your little ones into the ways you soothe them to sleep. As we've learned, temperament affects how well your babies are able to buffer input from their senses when needed, and this is directly linked to their ability to go to sleep and stay asleep.

Alert Babies and Sleep

If you find that you have an alert baby or two—a baby or babies who are much more sensitive to external (and internal) input—the usual sleep training advice doesn't always do the trick. Kim has found in her work with tens of thousands of families that an alert, intense, sensitive temperament may be the dividing line between a child who sleeps easily and one who takes a bit longer to learn.

Some babies react less strongly to stimuli and events, and generally stay on a fairly even keel. They are able to filter out a lot of the external noise and stimulation in order to turn toward sleep. Because alert babies have a much thinner barrier, sleep is more of a challenge. They are bombarded by sensory and other information and so have a lot more of it to manage. They need more help to shut the world out and go to sleep.

Kim has found that alert babies also tend to exhibit other traits that impact sleep and sleep shaping/coaching:

Intensity
When it comes to reactions, everything seems bigger with alert babies. If they're happy, they're *really* happy, and everyone is happy. Once they

get upset, they are *incredibly* upset, and so is everyone else. These are the babies whose parents say, "If I don't get to them in a few seconds, all bets are off." Intensity is the key trait that throws sleep training off track. These powerhouses don't just fuss for fifteen minutes then fall asleep; it can be an hour or more of hysterical crying, for many nights in a row, without any change. It's no wonder that parents of alert babies abandon the typical sleep coaching methods. It's also why the slowest and gentlest approaches of the Baby-Led Sleep Shaping and Coaching process work best for them.

Persistence

Easygoing and *flexible* are not in these babies' vocabularies; they do not give up easily on what they want and can often outlast you! I try to always gently remind parents that this trait is looked at very positively in the real world. But HOLY COW can it be frustrating when they are little. It's important to know that any time you try to change these babies' familiar patterns, they are going to fight you. Stay present, supportive, and consistent, and they will eventually accept the new pattern and settle in. Stay strong.

Perceptiveness

These babies notice *everything*! In the big picture, this can be a valuable skill, as they can grow into sensitive young adults who empathize easily with others. When it comes to sleep, however, their perceptiveness means you will need to be especially consistent. They will notice every small change in the routine or environment, and this can be unsettling to them. You need to have a routine that is clear and consistent.

Engagement

These babies have FOMO before they even know what FOMO means. They are harder to read in regard to sleep because they are always alert. They may not give off the same sleep cues as other babies, so it's important to watch the clock and not just their cues to avoid them getting overtired.

Irregularity and Unpredictability

Sometimes, these babies have no reliable pattern to their feeding, sleep, or activity. These babies do things differently every day. They may sleep well one night and not the next. You may try something that totally worked one day only to find out that it doesn't work the next. Now multiply that unpredictability by two! If this is what's going on in your house, you have to trust that what you are doing for their sleep will work in the long run—even if you don't see consistent results every night. Have a plan, stick to it, and your little ones will eventually (mostly) get on board.

Supporting Your Alert Baby

Alert babies prove just how much sleep and temperament are related. Intensity, persistence, sensitivity, and the other alert baby traits can create a perfect storm that not only makes sleep harder but also throws parents for a loop when it comes to sleep training. Many other sleep books will say that sleep training only takes three or four days of "some mild protest," but after two hours of sweating and pleading and crying, night after night with no improvement, parents of alert babies often give up and just rock them to sleep—convinced that maybe they just stink at parenting. Gang, it's not you. It's temperament. You are doing a great job. We just have to figure out a different way to handle things with alert babies.

 Twiniversity Tip

Reviewing your twinnies' sleep tracker regularly will help you understand how much sleep your alert baby or babies really need. Alert children often seem like they don't need as much sleep because their sleepy cues are not as obvious. Kim and I still suggest you try to get them the recommended hours of sleep for their age. It helps to make sure that they get quality sleep during their naps and have a consistent, early bedtime.

Alert children have their world filter wide open. It's our job to help them manage this large amount of input until they get old enough to begin to manage it on their own. It will take a few years, but keep in mind, they have only been humans for a few weeks now. The world is a lot to take in. Many adults still haven't figured out how to balance it all.

In the meantime, YOU are their filter, and it is your job to read their cues . . . even when your baby is harder to read. Stay curious and continue to SOAR!

If you find yourself struggling with your alert baby's or babies' sleep, you can use the QR code to reach out to Kim and her Sleep Coaches for more help.

 Getting You and Your Duo to Sleep

As you're learning about what's changing with your twinnies, you also should take a moment to look at how far you've come. I hope you're starting to notice that all the hard work you've been putting in by being your babies' detective and setting the stage for the best possible sleep is starting to pay off. If you're still struggling, take a breath. Rome wasn't built in a day, as the saying goes, and your twinnies will get the hang of it as long as you remain consistent.

Sleep Needs in Healthy Full-Term Babies

The typical sleep average for your baby in this third month is **ten hours at night and five hours during the day spread out over several naps** (three to four, or more if their naps are short). At night, you can expect your babies to wake two to three times, between 10 PM and 6 AM. Your babies can now be awake for up to one and a half to two hours at a time.

Night Sleep Consolidation Continues

At this point (we hope!), your twins are taking one extended stretch at night that typically begins after bedtime (you've learned about supporting this longer period with a dream feed). Before now, your infants were sleeping and waking to feed in intervals driven by their feeding needs. By this time, their circadian rhythms are now helping drive a regular nighttime stretch. This stretch, which you may have started to see at the end of last month, may average between **four and six hours**. Some babies may go a little longer, but it's rare.

As their circadian rhythms evolve, you can help them along by implementing some predictability in nighttime routines and bedtime. We will give you more tips for encouraging this long stretch! After this one long stretch, your babies will probably wake for a feeding every two to four hours for the rest of the night.

Napping

As always, we want to make sure that your kiddos are getting enough sleep during the day so that they are not overtired at bedtime. Night sleep continues to develop at this age, but daytime sleep is still kind of random, so any sleep shaping that you're doing should be focused on bedtime. Naps are all about filling that daytime sleep tank. We recommend getting your babies to sleep and getting them to stay asleep any way you can: in a dim or dark room at home, in a stroller or front carrier, while rocked to sleep and then held through their entire nap . . . whatever's necessary. As you are filling your twinnies' daytime sleep tanks, focus on keeping their wake windows short so they don't get overtired, particularly if you find that your kiddos are currently taking short naps.

Snack Naps

Nap lengths can vary greatly in these early months, and taking thirty- to forty-minute naps all day long is completely normal for this age. Yes, it would be great if your duo had hour and a half– to two-hour naps. However, this is not always in the cards, and that's OK.

Supporting Your Babies' Sleep

As your twins' circadian rhythms start to develop, nights begin to take shape. This is the first stage of sleep development and becomes the perfect time to nurture the basics of healthy sleep habits.

The Elements of Baby-Led Sleep Shaping (Month Three and Beyond)

1. Create a sleep-friendly environment for your duo, which should include:
   - Room-darkening shades.
   - Soothing colors.
   - White noise.
   - Cool temperature.
2. Create daily routines:
   - At bedtime, use a consistent, soothing routine. Do this in your twins' nursery if you plan to eventually transition them there, even if you are currently room sharing.
   - Create a shorter pre-nap version of your pre-bed routine.
3. Prevent overstimulation by following Kim's 3 PM Rule.
4. Don't let your twins sleep through daytime feedings (i.e., over three hours at a time).
5. Support your twins' budding circadian rhythms:
   - Watch their wake windows.
   - Dim lights at night.
   - Expose them to sunshine in the morning.
6. Regulate your twins' wake-up. For example, always wake them for the day at 7:30 AM.
7. Regulate your twins' bedtime. Note the time that they usually fall asleep for the night and consider setting that time as their bedtime.

8. Focus on creating one longer stretch of sleep at night. Try a dream feed to see if it helps (page 138).
9. Fill your twins' daytime sleep tanks:
   - Help them get naps any way you can: rocking, holding, pushing them in the stroller.
   - Watch for their sleepy cues and avoid letting them get overtired.
10. Begin to move bedtime earlier. Each night, move your babies' bedtime earlier by fifteen minutes until you are putting them down in their cribs between 7 and 8 PM. Bedtime should be no more than two hours after their last nap.

We've already suggested some sleep shaping steps in your twinnies' first two months. You'll learn more sleep shaping suggestions this month. These elements promote high-quality sleep and help support the lengthening of their first stretch of night sleep. They'll also help create a strong foundation for sleep coaching in the future.

Too Early for Sleep Training or Coaching

Parents are often afraid that they will create poor long-term sleep habits if they don't start sleep training their babies at three months (or even six weeks!). Don't worry. Your twins are not ready for sleep training or sleep coaching. In fact, when parents start too early, they often end up having to start the sleep coaching process all over again several months later because the training didn't take.

A baby at this age is not developmentally ready for sleep training or coaching; they don't yet have the skills to help them with the challenge of soothing themselves to sleep.

For now, bonding with your twins by reading their cues and responding accordingly is still your most important focus. At this stage, calming and soothing can actually help link sleep cycles and nurture your twins' circadian rhythms—so it plays a very important role in supporting both current and future sleep.

Moving Bedtime Earlier

Since night sleep develops first, our focus at this time is on bedtime and your kiddos' one long nighttime stretch. This is the first building block in shaping their sleep patterns.

Last month, you gently regulated your twins' wake time; now is the age to start regulating their bedtime, too. If your babies are waking up cranky from a late nap between 6 and 8 PM, then this is a sign to move their bedtime earlier. Then you'll want to work backward to calculate when to wake them from their last afternoon nap. If bedtime is around 7 PM, and your twins have a sixty- to ninety-minute wake window, then you'll want to wake them from their last afternoon nap no later than 5:30 PM.

If your twins' sleep time has not naturally moved earlier, you can help them along. Move their routine fifteen minutes *earlier* each night until you get to around 7 PM.

Why Is Bedtime So Early?

While it's perfectly OK for you to stay up until 10 PM, most babies are simply not capable of staying awake past 7 or 7:30 PM without getting a second wind (something you've likely experienced with them already!). Watch your twins for early sleepy signs, and start the bedtime routine as soon as you see those cues, if not before.

Why is it so important that your baby is not overtired at bedtime? Being awake too long (at any time during the day) causes elevated levels of cortisol, your primary stress hormone, which makes it more challenging to fall asleep and stay asleep. It also causes fragmented sleep cycles. When your babies become overtired, they have trouble falling asleep and staying asleep.

You may see the following with overtired babies:

- Difficulty falling asleep (often taking forty to sixty minutes).
- Steady crying at bedtime (even when comforted) that can last up to sixty minutes.
- Waking within an hour of going to bed and needing help falling back asleep.
- Additional night wakings.
- Restless sleep.

- Early morning rising (before 6 AM).
- Poor naps the next day—leading to poor sleep again the following night.

If you put your child to sleep earlier (around 7 PM), they will have an easier time settling into sleep and have less chance of night wakings and early rising. And you'll prevent them from falling into an overtired cycle.

No Playtime at Dream Time

Yes, your twinnies are the sweetest. I know you want to snuggle them. I know you missed them all day. I get it. They are delicious. BUT . . . they need to rest. If you keep them up so you can play with them after work until you are ready for them to go to sleep, odds are they'll be going to sleep way past the time they're ready to. And that's only going to make your night more difficult.

If you have no way around a late bedtime, however, listen to the Sleep Lady. Kim recommends making a late afternoon/early evening nap a priority so your twinnies can make it to a later bedtime without getting overtired. Kim has worked with a very small percentage of babies where they were able to do this successfully—but only when the parents diligently committed to filling their daytime sleep tank and prioritizing their late afternoon nap. Kim also ascribes some of this success to those babies' easy temperaments—which you have no control over. So, this may work, or it may not. Sorry to be the bearer of bad news!

Gentle Pre-Sleep Coaching Techniques: The Switcheroo and Jiggle and Soothe

Although your babies are too young for sleep coaching, if their sleep is going well and you would like to begin practicing something gentle that will get them *ready* for sleep coaching, we have a few options you can try. Note: We recommend you make these a team sport and not try them solo, at least for the first few bedtimes.

The Switcheroo is a very gentle technique you can try if you are heading back to work and need a solution for getting your duo down for naps. You can also try Jiggle and Soothe to help your twinnies become more adjusted to their sleep space, although—while it still falls under the Baby-Led Sleep Shaping (rather than Coaching) umbrella—it can feel like a bigger step.

Baby-Led Sleep Shaping and Coaching ™

The gentle approach led by your duos'
unique temperaments and needs

Caregivers soothe and assist less
as your duos' skills increase

Caregivers
put twins
to sleep
(day and
night)

Switcheroo

Jiggle and Soothe

Super Slow Shuffle
(for alert babies)

Jiggle and Soothe 2.0

Modified Shuffle

sleep shaping foundation

The Switcheroo with Twins

Your babies probably have a familiar way of being put to sleep, which they associate with going to sleep and need in order to do so—what's called a sleep crutch. If, for example, your babies are always nursed to sleep, that might be the only way they know how to fall asleep—which can make naps at daycare or with a nanny difficult, if not impossible.

Sleep crutches are VERY normal at this age! But what if you could gently switch your baby to a new way of going to sleep without going so far as sleep coaching (which your twins are not yet ready for)?

The Switcheroo is a small preparatory technique you can try to *switch* your babies' sleep associations. It expands their repertoire of ways to fall asleep, which is helpful—even critical—if you need another adult to put them to sleep (or if you're nursing and would like to get a break from nursing them to sleep)!

Let's say your twins are currently used to being nursed to sleep. To perform the Switcheroo, nurse them *almost* to sleep, then pass them off to another parent or caregiver (or two) who then rocks them to sleep completely before putting them down in their sleep space. Yes, you are creating a *new* sleep crutch—rocking—but at least this one doesn't require a nursing mama bear.

A similar switch is from nursing to bottle-feeding. You can follow your standard pre-sleep routine and then offer your twins bottles, so they can feed to sleep that way. Now you have babies who can be fed to sleep by a number of different caregivers.

An added benefit of the Switcheroo is that your twins will be less attached to whatever association you swap in because it is so new. This new association may be easier to drop than their original association when you are ready for sleep coaching in the future.

Remember, don't worry if you are using strategies such as nursing, rocking, or comforting one or both of your babies to sleep if it is what is working for you right now. These aren't necessarily bad habits, and they can easily be phased out when your kiddos are older and more capable of learning how to fall sleep independently.

THE JIGGLE AND SOOTHE WITH TWINS

If it feels like things are starting to fall into place in the sleep department and your babies may be ready for the next step, try Kim's Jiggle and Soothe. The Jiggle and Soothe is not a sleep coaching method, but it will help prepare your kiddos (and you) for Gentle Sleep Coaching in the next couple of months.

Why We Start at Bedtime (and Wait on the Rest of the Night)

Bedtime is the easiest time to sleep shape and sleep coach because, as darkness comes in the evening, it cues your twinnies' bodies to produce melatonin, which makes their bodies feel drowsy. This, plus the sleep pressure that has been building in their tiny bodies throughout the day, makes it easier for them to fall asleep.

Some families focus on sleep shaping and coaching only at bedtime for a long time. They do whatever they need to in the middle of the night (feeding, rocking, holding), and also during naps, so they get that crucial daytime sleep. What we want from this early bedtime sleep shaping is for your babies to make that little bit of progress that lets you say, "Oh! It's working!" so that you feel empowered and have faith in the process—and in your twinnies.

To practice the Jiggle and Soothe:

1. Put each baby down in their crib *already* asleep. This means that you can use whatever soothing methods you've been using (feeding, rocking, shushing, patting, etc.) to help your twinnies get there.
2. Once you lay your babies down in their sleep space, gently jiggle their chests a little bit. (Kim calls this "jiggling the burrito" because if your baby is still swaddled, they look like they are snuggly folded into a tortilla like a baby burrito.) The jiggling will cause your babies to wake a little, open their eyes, and hopefully recognize where they are (in their sleep space).

3. Pat and shush your babies to get them *back* to sleep.

4. If your babies wake fully or becomes upset, pick them up and comfort them back to sleep. (This is why we recommend having a partner! You can each pick up one of your babies if needed.)

5. Try again the next night to get them used to the process.

If your babies are responding particularly well to the Jiggle and Soothe, you're welcome to page ahead to "Your Twins' Fourth Month" and try some of the more advanced Baby-Led Sleep Shaping tips we share there. But again—don't worry if they are not yet ready!

Modifying the Baby-Led Sleep Techniques

If your twinnies aren't ready for the Switcheroo or the Jiggle and Soothe, it's OK. I don't want you to be brokenhearted if one or both of your twinnies aren't up to the task this month simply because you're reading about them in this month's chapter.

One option is to try breaking any technique we've suggested into multiple baby steps to make them very gradual. You can—and I might argue should (if I dare use that word—EEK!)—modify the methods to work for you and your twinnies. Modifications are part of the foundation of Baby-Led Sleep Shaping and Coaching. You always want to be led by your kiddos' unique temperaments and needs. Especially if your twins are a bit more alert than most, modifications will be the name of the game.

Sleep Challenges at This Age

You've read the sleep expectations for your twinnies at this age and know that your kiddos are still unlikely to sleep through the night this month. If you are struggling with your little ones, our main suggestions are to double down on our sleep shaping guidelines and try out either the Switcheroo or the Jiggle and Soothe. But there are a few other sleep challenges you may also be facing this month.

Not Seeing the Long Stretch at Bedtime

If you're not yet seeing that one longer stretch at night, please go back over the sleep shaping guidelines on page 167 to make sure that you've implemented each of them. These elements are specifically recommended to help your babies develop this longer stretch. Another solution is to try a dream feed. See the dream feed tip on page 156 earlier in this chapter.

Swaddle Weaning

 If your twins are not yet rolling, you can continue to swaddle them. If they *are* rolling, however, you'll want to wean them from the swaddle.

You can go cold turkey and just stop using the swaddle outright, or you can try a more gradual approach.

To gradually wean your babies from their swaddles, begin by wrapping them as you have been but leave one arm out. If it goes well with one arm, move to having both arms out and wrapping the swaddle around their chest to provide comfort. At this point you can also consider switching to a product like a sleep sack that allows your babies' arms to be free.

Whenever you make a change in your twins' sleep routine, you have to be prepared for them to be frustrated, upset, and cry a bit. Make sure you're making any change after a day of good naps and following their standard pre-sleep routine. If you have a sensitive baby who really likes the comfort of the swaddle, you might want to try the Switcheroo by holding them in the sleep sack until they fall asleep. Just be prepared for them to wake more frequently during this transition.

Taking Care of You

It may seem like you have no time for yourself lately, but that is exactly when making that time is most necessary. Here are a few key self-care recommendations for this month:

- Commit to having off-duty time each week like we suggested in chapter 1. Start small. Go for a walk by yourself. Grab a cup of coffee with a friend for thirty minutes. It doesn't have to be anything big.
- Take a moment to realize how awesome you are. You grew two humans in your body, they are here, and you're reading a book on how to help them sleep. You're a great parent, you look fantastic (I should have told you

that before—I meant to, I just had too much to tell you about sleep), and you're seriously doing great.

- Make sure you are getting your basic needs met. Are you sleeping, eating, staying connected enough?
- Do for you what you would do for others. If your bestie was sleeping as much as you are, if they were eating as well as you are, if they were staying connected to the people they love as much as you are, how would you feel they were doing? Would you think they need help?
- Check in with your partner. Are you communicating enough? Are you asking for what you need? Are they? Do you feel comfortable expressing how you feel about anything and everything? Do you feel judged? Do you feel understood and heard? Reconnect emotionally and maybe even physically, if you are up for it.
- Turn on a song and dance around the room with the twins as your audience. Dance parties are a STAPLE in the Diaz house. We had one every single Friday till the twins went to high school and had different schedules. Not only does a dance party help you celebrate having another week under your belt, it's also a great way to teach your twins some of your favorite songs, and soon enough, they will be teaching you some of theirs.

Buckle Up, Things Might Get Bumpy

There are positive changes coming ahead—but first, there's the four-month sleep regression. While it may feel challenging to support your baby through this phase, the result will be even better sleep in the future. Fear not, we'll help you navigate this stage in the next chapter!

FAST to Sleep Summary

Well, look at you! You've been learning the ropes this whole time, and now you know so much. This month, the big focus has been teaching you even more calming and soothing strategies, along with helping you identify your twinnies' ideal sleep schedule by reading their cues. You are doing so great! Take a moment to realize how far you've come and pat yourself on the back. You deserve it.

What to Focus on This Month

1. Aim for up to forty-five to sixty minutes of tummy time total per day spread across a few sessions. This is a great age for your twinnies to start interacting with each other and even some toys around them. It's so much fun to watch.

2. Remember, your duo may take only one long extended sleep stretch without eating in each twenty-four-hour period (assuming your doc is cool with their weights and how they are growing). Feeding them every two to three hours during the day will help to ensure this long stretch comes at night. That may mean waking your babies at that three-hour mark during the day if feeding time approaches and they are still asleep.

3. Put in place the Baby-Led Sleep Shaping elements (page 167), including beginning to move bedtime earlier. Read about the Switcheroo and Jiggle and Soothe to see if you want to try out either of these Baby-Led Sleep Shaping approaches with your twins.

4. Think of yourself a bit each day. Remember, self-care is not selfish. You need to take a moment for you, so you can be better for your crew.

What Not to Worry About

Nap coaching, night weaning, or sleep coaching. Your babies might not be ready yet!

For a printable PDF of this month's "FAST to Sleep Summary" plus helpful book bonuses, use the QR code.

Notes

chapter six

Your Twins' Fourth Month

Ages 12 Weeks to 16 Weeks

This month, you'll learn about the four-month sleep regression and what you can do to soothe your duo through this time. You'll also be introduced to the Baby-Led Sleep Coaching Readiness Checklist to see if your twins are ready for some gentle Baby-Led Sleep Coaching steps. If they are, we'll offer a few things you can try. (Remember to take adjusted age into consideration, especially when it comes to sleep.)

What Happened to My Baby?

I'm not crying, you're crying. They are growing up so fast! Where did the time go? Your twinnies are turning into real little people, right before your eyes. Can you believe it?

We have a little warning for you, though: This month may be a struggle. Hey, don't get mad at the messenger here. It's all thanks to the four-month sleep regression. For most families, it can feel like their kiddos are taking a step back when it comes to sleep, losing all the progress they had been making. It's OK. We understand. We've been there, done that, and, ahem . . . wrote the book on it! (I just high-fived myself.)

First, we'll help you to understand what your twins are going through, and second, we'll help you create the foundation for better sleep in the future—even if things are looking rough right now. With a little extra planning and tailored tools, your duo's response to this development stage doesn't have to turn your life (and sleep) upside down any longer than it takes your twinnies to get through it.

Your Developing Duo

Your twins are experiencing intense physical and neurological growth this month. Those consistent routines you worked so hard on last month and the month before may not work like they used to, and their sleep is likely to be disrupted. And this particular developmental phase can last longer than the previous ones—from one week all the way up to six weeks!

Changes in brain and body development tend to cause behavioral changes (including sleep changes), and this can—understandably—be very frustrating to parents! Plus, when parents aren't aware of what's developmentally going on with their kiddos, they can also get pretty worried.

Your babies are beginning to develop depth perception and will go through a burst of new cognitive awareness—they are starting to understand what is going on around them. Building on last month's development, this month brings increased senses of smell, sight, taste, hearing, and touch into their world.

At this point, your babies will start to make more intentional movements and sounds. They are able to see a toy that they want, reach for it, and grab it. They can then turn it around, pass it to their other hand, put it in their mouth, or pass it to their twinnie BFF. This is an especially helpful development if your babies are soothed by a pacifier. Although it won't happen this month, they will eventually be able to reach for a fallen pacifier and bring it back to their mouth on their own. Yay! On the safety side, however, you'll now have to keep a closer eye on their surroundings because they might grab something sharp or a hot cup of coffee without understanding the consequences.

Your babies might make more attempts to roll at this age. Maybe they have already succeeded and are trying to replicate the move, or maybe they are trying to do so for the very first time. Remember that rolling will be part of their sleep self-soothing toolbox. When they need to change positions, they'll be able to do so themselves rather than needing your help.

At this stage, babies have learned to push a bottle or breast away from their mouth when they are full. They can now use movement alongside their other cues to give you a better idea of what they are trying to communicate. You still need to keep your detective hat on! When your babies push a bottle or breast away, it could mean that they are full . . . or it could be that they are simply distracted. Your babies are more aware of their surroundings than ever and more easily distracted by them, too. Your babies will also start to recognize their own names around this time. Once they do, your communication with them really kicks into high gear!

According to *The Wonder Weeks*, your babies are now going through a major developmental leap, and as with other leaps, this explains their fussiness, moodiness, and clinginess. You may find them wanting more of your attention and cueing you for more touch, holding, and entertainment.

Yeah, this can be a struggle with two, but you'll figure it out. It's not safe to hold two and walk around, but you can always use two bouncy seats sitting on the floor, one on either side of you so you can have a hand on each and even rock them. When twins get clingy, it tends to quickly go from zero to sixty in the stress department. Start thinking of ways you can split yourself in two (like the bouncy chairs), or consider having a bit more help close at hand for those times you need all hands on deck!

Your twins are learning so many new things, like cause and effect and the beginning of object permanence (more on this next month!). They may use their voice to squeal, laugh, cough, or cry just to elicit a response from you. A smidge of shyness or anxiety about strangers may also begin to set in at this stage, and your babies may want to stay close to you and your partner. Even other family members such as grandparents or aunts and uncles may induce a meltdown when they leave the comfort and safety of your arms.

The Four-Month Sleep Regression (Insert Dramatic Music Here!)

Sometime between the fourteenth and seventeenth week, your babies may go through what is commonly called the *four-month sleep regression*, a period of unusually excessive fussiness and sleep disruption. Please keep in mind that not all babies experience this disruption. But our main focus for the month be helping navigate this change for parents whose babies do experience it.

The four-month sleep regression has two causes. The first is the physical and neurological developmental changes you just learned about. Anytime a baby experiences physical and neurological development, sleep is often disrupted because it makes it harder for them to *go* to sleep in the first place. These types of developmental changes also regularly cause extra fussiness and clinginess.

The second cause of sleep disruption this month is the way your twinnies' sleep cycles are changing. When your twins were first born, they spent equal time in REM sleep and non-REM sleep. This month they are beginning to enter the adult world of sleep, which means that, instead of going from just one sleep stage (REM sleep) to a second (deep sleep), they will start cycling through four very distinct sleep stages, just like you: two light stages of sleep, deep sleep, and REM sleep. In the past, your twinnies might have been a bit restless at the beginning of each sleep cycle, but once they transitioned into their non-REM sleep stage, they slept soundly. Now, they are beginning to wake *between* sleep stages.

The problem is that our kiddos are not yet used to this new sleep cycle, and to those more frequent wakings. Your babies also still have the Moro (or startle) reflex that they gained at birth, so when they enter active sleep during each sleep cycle, they can find themselves startling, which wakes them further. And whereas before, when they woke, they might have still been drowsy and able to get back to sleep easily on their own, now they are waking *completely*, because they are more aware of their environment. If they don't know how to get back to sleep on their own, they look for someone who can help: a parent or caregiver.

As if that wasn't enough, your twins actually get most of their deep sleep at the beginning of the night during that one extended stretch. So, while they may start the night sleeping five hours straight, they will then begin to wake at regular intervals later in the night. Oh, joy (she says sarcastically).

Supporting Development for Better Sleep

Physical and neurological developments get your babies closer to being able to soothe themselves and learn to sleep better on their own. Helping them with their physical development at this age gets them closer to being able to self-soothe, which will help them get themselves both to sleep at bedtime and back to sleep when they wake at night.

Tummy Time

In month four, your babies can handle *up to ninety minutes of tummy time a day, broken out into several sessions.*

Sometimes both parents and babies are sick of tummy time by this month. Gentle reminder: Tummy time is really important! Putting our babies in a position they don't normally find themselves builds muscles and lets our babies learn skills that will help them later learn to roll, crawl, and eventually walk.

Your babies might feel uncomfortable and get frustrated during tummy time. Some babies really let you know that they DON'T LIKE TUMMY TIME! It's tempting to give them a pass and skip it for the day. But while your duo might not like what is happening at the moment, it will help them in the long run.

This is a good opportunity to reframe the tummy time experience as one of many dances you will do with your twins where you let them feel a little frustration. When they fuss, rather than immediately ending the session, you can put a light hand on their back and verbally console them so that they know you are there and supporting them. You can say, "Yes, I'm sure this feels frustrating. You're not used to being in this position, are you? But you're not alone. I'm here with you and so is your brother/sister." As we reassure them, we can count to twenty to lengthen tummy time just a little, while also reassuring our babies through this frustrating moment. You will go through something similar as you engage in the Baby-Led Sleep Coaching steps.

One of the first signs that tummy time is working is when your baby rolls over on their own. That is what you are all working toward!

Remember you can put your twinnies head-to-head or side to side, remembering to rotate them from time to time so they can work on different muscles. The squeals of their brother or sister will be another entertaining aspect to their baby workout time.

As always, when deciding when to have some tummy time, pick times when your babies are alert, aware, and social (but not right after feeding so they are less likely to spit up).

 ## Twiniversity Tip

If you suspect that one or both of your twinnies may be falling behind in some skills, speak to your pediatrician about it. If they are only slightly behind on their milestones, the doc will probably tell you not to worry—but if you still are, you have the right to get an evaluation with or without your provider's  approval. Most states have an early intervention program in which trained specialists are available to evaluate whether one or both of your kids could use a little extra tutoring, so to speak. This could be with physical development, fine motor development, or even speech and feeding development. To find out more about early intervention, use the QR code.

 ## Feeding

Feeding may seem to regress this month, along with sleep. Your babies may be more distracted while feeding in the daytime due to their increased awareness of their surroundings. They may have shorter, more frequent feeds and need additional feeds at night when going through this stage. While the latter is often due to them feeding less during the day, they may also just need more calories for growth and development. With all the changes in feeding and sleep, it may feel like you have gone back to the newborn stage! But remember, it's just a phase.

Feeding at This Age

On average, babies feed ***every two and a half to three hours (some up to four hours) during the day*** and may go one long stretch (between four and six hours) without eating at night. By the end of this month, some babies can—with your doctor's permission—take an eight-hour stretch of sleep without feeding. They will take in ***between four and six ounces per feeding***.

Feeding amounts will depend on how long your babies sleep at night and how frequently they eat during the day. If they reduce their feedings at night, they may need to feed more during the day, and if they reduce their feedings during the day—whether due to developmental milestones, distraction, starting daycare, or transitioning to a bottle—they may need to feed more at night.

A possible shift in appetite as a result of the four-month developmental milestones may cause nursing mamas to experience a drop in milk supply. If you experience this, you can add an evening dream feed before you go to bed to make sure your babies are getting enough milk and try to get that nice long stretch of sleep together with your twinnies. You might want to add a power pumping session in as well (see the QR code for more information).

This month, we've added naps to our sample schedule. Below is a typical four-hour feeding cycle; if you need to stay on a three-hour feeding cycle, please refer back to previous months' sample schedules. And remember, this is just a sample! Your twinnies' daily schedule can look different from the one we have here.

For your own printable copy of this schedule, see the QR code.

The Myth of Solids, Formula, and Sleep

Parents regularly ask if offering their babies solids now will help them sleep better at night. The answer is that research doesn't support the idea that solids promote better nighttime sleep. A study in the *New England Journal of Medicine* found that feeding rice cereal to babies before six months of age did not help them sleep longer. In fact, it found that babies who were fed rice cereal before four months of age slept *less*.

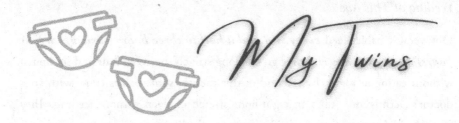

Fourth Month Home Daily Schedule

Sample Schedule Based on 4hr Feedings*

6am		6pm	🦆 📖
7am	🩲 🍼	7pm	🩲 🍼 🛏️zzZ
8am	🎠	8pm	
9am	zzZ ☕	9pm	☕
10am	🚼 🎠	10pm	
11am	🩲 🍼	11pm	🩲 🍼
12pm	🎠	12am	
1pm	zzZ	1am	
2pm	🎠 ☕	2am	
3pm	🩲 🍼	3am	🩲 🍼
4pm	🎠	4am	
5pm	zzZ	5am	

🩲 Diaper change	🚼 Go outside	zzZ Bed time	📖 Read
🍼 Feed breast/bottle	zzZ Naptime	🦆 Bath	🎠 Play time
	☕ Take a moment		

*Always check with your doc about schedule specifics
for your particular twins

The myth that feeding your baby solids will help them sleep longer at night persists because sometimes it does work—just not for the reason you think. If a baby is distracted and not eating well during the day, then they don't feel full at night, and this can impact sleep. Sometimes, if they are given a bottle with rice at night, they might sleep longer. But the real issue is that they are not getting enough milk or formula during the day. Cereal is also linked to obesity in babies— another reason to manage the real issue of low feeding during the day, rather than try to treat the symptoms with solids.

As I've said before, both Kim and I discourage parents from starting solids simply for sleep reasons. At this age, breast milk and formula are still your twinnies' best source of nutrition. To determine the best time to start on solids, speak with your pediatrician.

Supporting Sleep Through Feeding

As you support your twins through the four-month sleep regression, think of feeding as something you can adjust to encourage the sleep that they *are* getting.

Supporting Nighttime Feedings

At this age, it is completely normal for your babies to be waking during the night for one to three feedings between bedtime and morning. Don't be discouraged if you find one or both of your babies, who used to be able to sleep a longer stretch, all of a sudden begin waking more to feed—even if they were previously going six to eight hours without. They are growing rapidly and experiencing a developmental milestone, so they really DO need to eat. (That said, we do want to help you get back that long stretch at night, and we also want to keep your twins from slipping into reverse cycling—more on that soon.)

Soon enough, you will miss those quiet night feedings. For real. You will. Don't believe me? It's OK. I'll be telling you "I told you so" before you know it.

As long as your twins are still eating during the night, it's important to maintain a sleep-friendly environment. During night feedings, make sure that you keep the room quiet and dark and cause as little disruption as possible. Doing this will gently remind them that nighttime is for sleep, not play.

You'll know if your kiddos need to feed at night by sharing your feeding log with your pediatrician and lactation consultant. If your twins are not hungry in the morning, then you can work on reducing their nighttime feedings. Just snacking when they wake in the middle of the night, instead of taking a full feed, can also be a sign that night feedings are no longer necessary—or can at least be reduced.

If your twins are not hungry in the morning, and you find they are sleeping in a bit longer, it might also be a sign that they are ready for some Gentle Sleep Coaching at night. Longer stretches of sleep are a great indicator that their tiny tummies are keeping them satisfied longer. Woohoo! (Check out the Baby-Led Sleep Coaching Readiness Checklist in the "Sleep" section of this chapter to read more about how and when to start.)

Not Seeing a Long Stretch of Sleep? Try a Dream Feed

If you have not yet seen this long stretch we've talked about, remember, a dream feed might help. A dream feed can help to reset the clock, stretching out the time before their next feed and making that their *long* stretch of the night.

If you put your babies to sleep at 7 PM, wake them slightly to feed them— without waking them fully—before you go to bed or just before they usually wake, for example at 9:45 PM. Do this for three to seven nights and see if a longer stretch of sleep occurs afterward. If it does, keep it up! If it doesn't, you'll need to try something else to get that long stretch.

For more on dream feeds, see "Your Twins' Second Month," page 138.

What Did I Do Wrong?

If you find yourself confused because last month you were seeing a long stretch of sleep, but now, with the four-month sleep regression, it's gone, please hold tight until you feel that the sleep regression has passed. Then check out the "Sleep" section of this month for how to bring the long stretch back.

Feeding Challenges in the Fourth Month

If you and your pediatrician haven't diagnosed or addressed a lingering feeding challenge or challenges, this would be the time to do so. You'll want to make sure that their feeding is on track before practicing the Baby-Led Sleep Coaching that we recommend at the end of this chapter and in the next.

Reverse Cycling

You learned about reverse cycling last month. If you suspect that your little ones are starting to reverse cycle, please return to "Your Twins' Third Month," page 159, to get tips on how to prevent it from continuing.

 ## Attachment

Your main job this month is soothing your babies through the four-month sleep regression. While you're doing this, you can continue to build attachment through daily and nightly routines and lots of snuggles and reassurance. The strong attachment and trust you've built over the last three months, and continue to reinforce this month, will help Baby-Led Sleep Shaping and Coaching go more smoothly in the near future.

 ## Soothing

When it comes to soothing your bitty beasts, do whatever you've found that works to get you through the four-month sleep regression. You will get through this! Use the tools we've shared the last four months, and keep an eye out for any new cues from your twinnies that tell you they could use some soothing. Have you noticed that they are starting to communicate through facial expressions? Yup, it's making for some great pictures, but it also means that their needs are getting easier and easier to figure out.

You may have noticed that your babies are becoming more sensitive, so soothing them effectively may require less intervention at this stage, instead of more. As they experience the fussiness that comes with their development this month, try out different levels of soothing to see what works best. Don't be surprised if your old tricks aren't working. Just keep trying new things. You've got this!

Soothing and Sleep

Because your twins' senses are more fine-tuned, you may need to make some changes to create a more soothing, sleep-friendly environment. You may have to use room-darkening shades and set the room at a lower temperature. If you are room sharing, you may need to move their cribs farther away from your bedside, since they are now more aware of your presence.

Your soothing pre-bed routine will continue to be important. You can use some of the soothing techniques we've recommended over the previous months: a warm bath (not necessary every night), massage, a book, rocking, patting, cuddling, and white noise. By this time, your babies can recognize repetition in their daily routine, so following your chosen routine and ending with a predictable bedtime can help them associate sleep with the routine. You can use a condensed version of this routine pre-nap.

This is a time to pay particular attention to their sleepy cues so that you can respond to them as quickly as possible. Your twins still need a nap every one to two hours (shorter naps will mean shorter wakeful windows), even if they are fighting it. Remember, if your babies are overtired, they will be more difficult to soothe and get to sleep.

Pacifiers This Month

By this age, you will probably have determined whether your kiddos seem soothed by a pacifier. In some cases, they may not be interested in using one, even if you wish they would.

If you are using one, we recommend using them for naps and nights only. Your twins have started to babble and make noises with their mouth, and you'll want to encourage this because it leads to even better communication. Keeping a pacifier in their mouths constantly prevents this much-needed verbalization practice. For more information about pacifiers, please see Months One and Two (pages 77 and 128).

Pacifiers and Sleep

Pacifiers are a blessing and a curse. Sure, they are a helpful tool to help your kiddos soothe themself, but babies at this age aren't able to control a pacifier on their own. That translates into you having to go help them pop those pacifiers back in when they wake up at night. Don't be shocked if you find yourself getting all your steps in at night running back and forth into their room every hour.

If you recognize yourself in that last paragraph, you have a couple of choices. You can:

- Purchase a pacifier-holding product, like a small stuffed animal that's attached to the pacifier, to make the pacifier easier for your child to retrieve.
- Say adios to the pacifier and have them get used to sucking on their own hands.

Pacifier Weaning

Some babies, particularly those who exhibit colic or reflux, become attached to sucking on something and might find it difficult to self-soothe any other way. This is the earliest age that your babies begin self-regulation, so they may not be ready to do this on their own. In this case, you may want them to keep using the pacifier (in which case you might need to replug their pacifier at night or use a pacifier-holding product).

If you *are* looking to wean your baby off using pacifiers for sleep, we recommend coming up with a solid sleep coaching plan (more on this in the "Getting You and Your Duo to Sleep" section on page 198) and starting at bedtime after your regular routine. A few options:

- You can let your babies suck on a pacifier as they fall asleep and then remove it *before* they are completely asleep. You can then pat and shush them to see if they continue the process of going to sleep without the pacifier.
- If your babies are particularly attached to a pacifier, you may find that you can get them used to going to sleep without it by starting with two minutes of patting and shushing before giving them the pacifier for the night,

and then increasing the patting and shushing by two minutes each night, to see if they will go to sleep without it.

- If your babies are particularly upset, you can even pick them up and rock them to sleep.

With a plan, many babies wean from the pacifier within two or three days. If you're finding that your baby is particularly upset when you try to put them to sleep without the pacifier but you want to stick with it, you can stretch the process of patting and shushing them before giving them the pacifier over a few weeks. If you are uncomfortable with the amount of crying at this time, you can halt the process and try it again in a few weeks, when their self-soothing capabilities are better developed.

Your Twinnies' Blossoming Self-Soothing Skills

Up to this point, you've provided soothing to your duo so that they can understand the difference between being regulated and dysregulated. Around this age, your kiddos become capable of very basic self-soothing. They may not be able to completely calm themselves down yet, but they are experimenting and may even be able to put themselves back to sleep using their new skills.

You can start to watch for signs of self-soothing as early as four months. Examples include:

- Rolling.
- Kicking.
- Raising and dropping their legs.
- Squeezing their legs together.
- Rubbing their head back and forth on a surface.
- Using a small attachment object.
- Sucking on their hands.
- Moving their hands to their body's midline to activate a calming response (they'll move their hands to their chest as adults do when we cross our arms).

While you might be able to see these new self-soothing skills during the day, your twins will also begin to apply them to the "going to sleep" process. This is great news, since sleeping longer stretches at night is dependent upon their ability to soothe themselves back to sleep when they wake up. We'll talk about this in more detail later in the chapter.

Reminder: If Your Twinnies Have Started Rolling, They Can No Longer Be Swaddled

You want your babies to learn to roll, but once they do, it means that swaddling is no longer an option for soothing. If your babies roll onto their stomach, they will need their arms free to roll to their back again. (It's OK if they don't roll yet at this stage, and it is highly likely that your babies have learned to roll one way but not the other.) Check out our suggestions in "Your Twins' Third Month" (page 175) for how to wean your kiddos from the swaddle.

SOAR for Soothing

As you learned earlier in this chapter, what worked last month to soothe your tiny team might not work this month, given the developmental changes they're experiencing. You may have to work even harder, as their detective, to figure out how to help.

When they start to get fussy, and your usual soothing techniques don't calm them, take a step back and follow the SOAR process (page 12). Keep in mind that, even though they might be fussier right now because of the four-month leap, they are learning new skills this month (like moving their hands to the middle of their body, sucking their hands and fingers, and rolling) that will soon help them better soothe themselves when they get upset. In the meantime, you can view these skills as another way they can ask for what they want and need.

Your babies will move through this fussy period. Hang in there!

Keep It Together

The four-month sleep regression can be a *challenging* time for parents, to put it nicely. Your job is to soothe your babies at a point when they are particularly difficult to soothe. If you find that your kiddos are starting to lose their tiny little minds, crying and pretty much having a full-on blowout, take a breath and keep it together.

No one said having twins was going to be easy, but you can do this, even on those difficult days when you feel like you've taken six steps back from a previous one step forward. Focus on your wins and try to stay positive. If you lose your cool, you'll get nowhere fast.

If you need a moment to breathe, take it. It's OK to be overwhelmed! But then you have to roll your sleeves up and get right back into your day. Step-by-step, you'll figure it out, I promise.

Soothing Challenges in the Fourth Month

Most of what you'll deal with on the soothing front this month has to do with your duo's changing preferences around soothing. Just keep experimenting to find something that works! I feel crappy saying that—it feels like a cop-out—but there is no quick fix. You really have to experiment based on each baby's temperament and preferred past soothing style. Never forget that this is just a phase. It WILL be over before you know it.

Colic versus GERD

Were your twins fussy and difficult to soothe in previous months, and you labeled this fussiness "colic"? If they are still exhibiting excessive fussiness, chances are they have GERD or other belly upsets. Check out "Your Twins' Second Month" and "Your Twins' Third Month" (pages 121 and 161) for symptoms and soothing solutions. You'll want to get your pediatrician involved as well and rule out food sensitivities and allergies.

Teething

If your twins are particularly fussy as you try to soothe them for sleep, you may want to determine if they are teething. If you think one or both are teething, you can wash your hands and push your finger on their lower front gums—if they cry out, you'll know you have a teether!

Most babies begin to get their primary teeth after the age of four months—usually between six and nine months. (Fun fact: If both parents got their teeth early, then the baby is likely to as well!) But the process of teething starts earlier, between three and six months. You may see your babies begin to drool at this time, because teething produces a lot of saliva, and they don't yet have the swallowing reflex to take care of it.

As their first teeth start to pop through their lower gum, the area starts to swell, and sucking can make swollen gums feel even worse. This means that if your usual go-to for soothing is a pacifier or nursing, these might not currently help.

You can instead freeze some formula or breast milk, pop it into a mesh bag, and ta-da! A teething relief treat. For more teething tricks, use the QR code.

Temperament

Most temperament research suggests that we only begin to see our children's temperaments at about four months of age. But there are many parents who say they could tell their baby's temperament in the delivery room! That's why we've been discussing this since the very beginning. If you feel as if you haven't yet seen one or both of babies' temperaments emerge already, it is likely that you will start seeing it now. And if you have seen it in the past, these days you are probably seeing it even more clearly.

As you know, understanding your twins' temperaments helps you know how to soothe them; what helps one baby in their fourth month might not help your other baby in their fourth month. But it will also help you know when, and how fast, to sleep coach. By paying attention to your babies' temperaments, you'll be able to set realistic goals and select the best sleep strategies from our sleep shaping and sleep coaching sections to support the overall success of your sleep coaching plan.

The Three Baby Temperaments

To better understand the connection between temperament and sleep, let's take a quick look at the results of a landmark study from 1956. The study found that 65 percent of babies fit easily into one of three distinct categories:

The Easy or Flexible Baby (40 percent of babies)

- Easygoing and adaptable.
- Adjusts easily to new situations.
- Quickly adjusts to routines.
- Regular sleeping and eating patterns.
- Easy to calm.
- Social, cheerful, and in a pleasant mood most of the time.

The Slow-to-Warm or Shy/Cautious Baby (15 percent of babies)

- Sensitive, cautious, and shy.
- May be difficult to soothe and care for at first but becomes easier over time.
- Prefers order and predictability.
- Thoughtful.
- Sensitive to new experiences.
- Needs more transition time to move comfortably between activities.

The Active/Fussy or Difficult Baby (What Kim Calls Alert) (10 percent of babies)

- Slow to adjust and adapt to change.
- Intense, demanding, and moody most of the time.
- Unpredictable and irregular feeding and sleeping patterns.
- Difficulty with new places, situations, and people.
- Intense reactions—willful, obstinate, needs THEIR way!
- Super sensitive and easily frustrated.
- Extremely active and physical.
- Needs constant attention.
- Determined and resourceful.

Easy babies historically do well with most sleep strategies because they are flexible and quick to adapt to new routines. You can usually move through the sleep coaching process without too many hiccups.

Slow-to-warm babies need more time to adapt to changes and transition into new routines. You may need to slow down the sleep coaching process for them and initially offer more soothing as you go along. For instance, your baby may need a pre-bed routine that is longer and slower than your other baby's. Results might seem to come a little bit slower than with easy babies, too. You may first see small changes in their sleep patterns within three or four days, instead of just one or two.

Active/Fussy (alert) babies need a lot more soothing and will move even slower through changes and new routines. Often, parents of these babies start with the simple step of committing to a regulated bedtime. Even with a lot of effort on their part, they may find improvement to their baby's sleep emerges very slowly. Eventually, when they get to sleep coaching, it requires *a lot of patience* on the part of the parents—both because the process is slower and because the results appear at a slower rate.

Alert babies do NOT do well with anything close to the Cry It Out method. They're easily dysregulated and usually difficult to calm down. These babies are often more persistent and will cry longer. They will try you! Don't be surprised when they hold out until they get what they want (for example, an easier, more comfortable way to fall asleep, like nursing or in your arms). These babies can sometimes also develop an aversion to their own crib if not well soothed. Yup, you read that correctly. Reacting quickly with soothing is your number one goal. You ideally want to calm your alert baby and their environment before putting them into their cribs because the calmer they are throughout the process, the easier it will be for them to actually *learn* how to self-soothe and go to sleep on their own.

When to Sleep Coach Alert Babies

Kim and I recommend that you consider waiting to start sleep coaching with these alert kiddos until around six months. Ugh, right? I know that's totally not what you wanted to hear (or read, in this case), but it might be your best option. The longer you wait, the more tools your alert baby or babies have to help themself fall asleep on their own.

Getting You and Your Duo to Sleep

You had the schedule down. Your babies were FINALLY sleeping better . . . and then, BAM! Suddenly all heck has broken loose.

What else can you do to support them (and yourself) through the four-month sleep regression? And what can you do afterward to get their sleep back on track?

Sleep Needs in Healthy Full-Term Babies

The typical sleep average for your twins in their fourth month is ***ten to eleven hours at night and four or five hours during the day, spread out over several naps.***

Time to Clean Your Wake Windows!

This month, you'll be able to use your understanding of your babies' wake windows—the length of time your kiddos can comfortably be awake before they get fussy—to regulate their nap times a little bit.

At this age, your kiddos' wake window length is a maximum of two hours, based on their current development. But remember, the wake window length we give each month is *just an average*, so you'll still want to watch your twins for sleepy cues to make sure they don't get tired earlier. Babies who are taking shorter naps may have a shorter wake window. It's OK if your babies are taking shorter naps—just get more naps in each a day, so they are well rested for bedtime.

Getting You Through the Four-Month Sleep Regression

While all developmental leaps can contribute to disrupted sleep, the one your kiddos are going through at four months is particularly disruptive because, as you'll remember from the development section, it's *related* to sleep. Your twins' sleep cycles are changing in a way that makes it harder for them to stay asleep.

While some babies breeze through this time of big ol' neurological and physical development, others find their sleep particularly wrecked and become pretty fussy. The most important thing to remember this month is that these are very normal reactions to the changes they are experiencing. The expectations you have for your twinnies' sleep may have to be temporarily thrown out the window.

This is a good time to observe your kiddos and give them a little space to figure out what may soothe them for sleepy time. Don't forget—it's normal for their needs to change. Soothing routines like rocking them might no longer work. Often parents panic and try to do too much to try to soothe their kiddos as their preferences are changing, and this can actually make things worse. They may need a little less of one thing or something completely different. They still need your help regulating themselves, but pulling back a bit can help you and them find out what is working and what's not.

Even though sleep itself is the "problem," when it comes to the four-month sleep regression, there are still a few things you can do to support your two through this time.

First, we recommend that you review all the Baby-Led Sleep Shaping steps we've recommended so far. Many of them will still work well in helping keep your twins' sleep from getting completely off track.

The Elements of Baby-Led Sleep Shaping (Month Three and Beyond)

1. Create a sleep-friendly environment for your duo, which should include:
   - Room-darkening shades.
   - Soothing colors.
   - White noise.
   - Cool temperature.
2. Create daily routines:
   - At bedtime, use a consistent, soothing routine. Do this in your twins' nursery if you plan to eventually transition them there, even if you are currently room sharing.
   - Create a shorter pre-nap version of your pre-bed routine.

3. Prevent overstimulation by following Kim's 3 PM Rule.

4. Don't let your twins sleep through daytime feedings (i.e., over three hours at a time).

5. Support your twins' budding circadian rhythms:
   - Watch their wake windows.
   - Dim lights at night.
   - Expose them to sunshine in the morning.

6. Regulate your twins' wake-up. For example, always wake them for the day at 7:30 AM.

7. Regulate your twins' bedtime. Note the time that they usually fall asleep for the night and consider setting that time as their bedtime.

8. Focus on creating one longer stretch of sleep at night. Try a dream feed to see if it helps (page 138).

9. Fill your twins' daytime sleep tanks:
   - Help them get naps any way you can: rocking, holding, pushing them in the stroller.
   - Watch for their sleepy cues and avoid letting them get overtired.

10. Begin to move bedtime earlier. Each night, move your babies' bedtime earlier by fifteen minutes until you are putting them down in their cribs between 7 and 8 PM. Bedtime should be no more than two hours after their last nap.

Second, you can add extra feedings or extra soothing to your routines during this time. Don't worry about creating bad habits with these additions! We will help you get back on track once your babies are through the regression.

Making Sure Wake-Ups and Bedtime Are Regulated

As parents struggle with babies whose sleep is disrupted this month, we find that they sometimes forget to stick with the sleep shaping pieces they previously had in place—especially regulating wake-ups and bedtime.

At this stage:

- Your babies' *wake time* should be between 6 AM and 7:30 AM.
- Your babies' *bedtime* should be between 6:30 PM and 7:30 PM.

When adults need help with their sleep, the first recommendation they are given is to regulate their bedtime and their wake time because this helps get their circadian rhythm in check. This works for babies as well!

For more on regulating your babies' wake time, please see "Your Twins' Second Month," page 115.

Twin Tweak

If you feel like one twinnie tends to need more sleep than the other, or needs a different bedtime or wake time, you can vary bedtime and wake time—but try to keep any discrepancies to thirty minutes *max* to keep everyone as close to the same schedule as possible. Gentle reminder: Your babies may have slightly different sleep needs, and that's OK. It can be an amazing opportunity for some one-on-one time with one of your babies.

Napping

Your goal for this month is to fill your babies' daytime sleep tanks any way you can so that even if they wake a lot at night during this regression, they are still getting enough sleep in each twenty-four-hour period. This means you can let your babies sleep on a walk in the stroller, in a carrier, or anywhere else they are safe and happy to sleep.

Am I Creating "Bad" Habits?

The four-month sleep regression is draining for Every! Single! Person! in the house. It's not surprising that, in your attempts to get your twinnies to sleep, you may feel like you've created what some folks would consider bad habits. You may be relying on methods like rocking them to sleep that work for now but that you definitely do not want to be using for the next couple of years.

You know what? That's OK! Habits can be changed once your twins are through this milestone and more capable of self-soothing. Do what you have to do to fill that daytime sleep tank in the meantime.

Once You've Made It Through the Regression

Are your babies starting to sleep better again? Do you see that one long stretch re-emerging at the beginning of the night? Do your twinnies seem less clingy and fussy? Even if only one kiddo has started showing signs of improvement (hey, we will take what we can get!), congratulations—you've made it through the four-month sleep regression! CELEBRATE! This is a huge step for not only them but you, too. Congrats!

While we encourage parents to double down on our Baby-Led Sleep Shaping elements during the four-month regression, we know that you may have taken a few detours to get your kiddos to sleep any way you could. So, as you all come out of the regression, your first step is to go back and make sure that *each of the sleep shaping elements is in place* (page 199). Getting back to a regular rhythm during both day and night will not only help their sleep but also let you assess if they are ready for Baby-Led Sleep Coaching.

Readjusting Your Twinnies' Internal Clocks

Now that you are on the other side of the four-month sleep regression, you may start to see your twins' routine re-establish and their sleeping and feeding schedules get back on track. To really make sure this sticks, it's important to get those kiddos out into the sunlight. Take them for walks, open the windows, or (if it's warm enough) have some tummy time on a blanket outside. Getting outside is critical for you, too (weather permitting, of course). Just thirty minutes in the morning and maybe even another thirty in the afternoon will help readjust their little internal clocks, especially if their sleep was particularly disrupted. For more on supporting your twins' circadian rhythms, please see "Your Twins' Third Month," page 150.

Twiniversity Tip

If you live in a super-cold or super-hot area and getting outside is impossible, try at least to open your shades and let the sunshine in! That giant ball of heat in the sky is one of our bodies' main sources of vitamin D. Grabbing a few rays of sunshine is great for your physical and emotional well-being. Also, studies show that a lack of vitamin D can raise chances of shorter sleep durations in children and adults. Soak it all in!

Reducing Night Feeds

After you've re-established any sleep shaping elements that fell by the wayside, it's important to make sure that your kiddos' feedings are going well during the day. Then, if you added a feeding, dream or otherwise, during their sleep regression, you may now be looking to wean them from it.

You'll want to do this gradually. One option is to slowly reduce—over the course of a few nights—the number of ounces you put in their bottles or the number of minutes they spend at the breast.

For example, if your babies are getting a dream feed before midnight, consider reducing the time they are feeding by one or two minutes (if breastfeeding) or the amount they are eating by a half to one ounce (if bottle-feeding) each night. You can do that over the course of a week. Once your babies get down to a two-minute nursing session or a two-ounce bottle, you can get rid of the feeding entirely.

Please be aware that weaning off one feed may slightly shift the timing of their next one. If you choose to keep the dream feed because the timing works better for you—then that is cool, too.

Weaning Already?

Talk with your doctor (and lactation consultant, if you are breastfeeding) to find out what night feedings should look like for your kiddos. Can they be weaned? How many feedings should be continued at this age? And if you aren't comfortable with their recommendations, don't hesitate to speak up. Everyone on Team Twinnie wants what's best for you and them!

Evaluating Your Twins' Readiness for Sleep Coaching

Now that the regression has passed, it's tempting to start sleep coaching right away. But while some babies may be ready for sleep coaching by four or five months of age, Kim has found that, generally, waiting until six months will bring you results faster and cause you less frustration. And at a minimum, we recommend that you don't consider sleep coaching until your babies have gone through the four-month sleep regression.

The absolute best time to teach your babies positive long-term sleep habits is after their brains and central nervous systems have matured, and this usually takes until a baby is six months old (adjusted age). Many other experts agree that six to eight months is the perfect window to work gently with a baby to teach them healthy sleep habits and self-soothing skills. Trust your gut—remember, you are your twinnies' expert.

CAN YOU SLEEP COACH EARLY?

As you might remember from the introduction, babies who are sleep coached too early can actually take longer to learn the skills necessary to get the rest they need. They are also more likely to cry longer and harder without showing signs of self-soothing. It is always better for your twinnies if you wait until they are developmentally capable of learning to self-soothe. For now, focus on sleep shaping first, especially if you haven't been already.

Don't rush the sleep coaching process! Starting it too early will not help anyone, and can lead to frustration and aggravation on your end. Who needs that? You have enough to worry about. Sleep shape before you sleep coach and you'll all be sleeping like babies before you know it.

The Case Against Cry It Out

If you've read the introduction, you know how I feel about the Cry It Out method, despite using it myself in the past. Even when I believed it was necessary, it was torture. With my alert Baby A, it took way too long and caused me significantly more stress than waking up all night. I wish I could turn back the hands of time and do it differently.

For years, the twin world led me to believe that the best way to get twins to sleep was to let them cry it out. But, as I always say, you don't know what you don't know. Learning about Kim's Gentle Sleep Coaching method really opened my eyes and made me realize that there was a better way. I knew that the twin world had to do better.

Babies are incapable of self-soothing themselves out of intense crying. And on top of that, intense crying means that they are dysregulated and not in a state to learn something new.

Macall Gordon puts it beautifully, saying, "The notion that learning is taking place when babies are hysterical just doesn't make sense. We want to nudge children into better patterns, not throw them into the deep end. Stepping in to help them manage big feelings is in our parent job description. It's no different with sleep."

Baby-Led Sleep Shaping and Coaching is effective because you are gently nudging your twins into new patterns when they are ready—following their lead, rather than pushing them to do something that is outside their capabilities.

Baby-Led Sleep Coaching Readiness Checklist

If you want to know if your babies are ready for Baby-Led Sleep Coaching—the next step in their learning—take a look at the following checklist. But please know that there is nothing wrong with your baby or babies if they are not yet ready. It's also OK to think they are ready only to find that they are not. You can always stop, wait a month or so, and try again.

Your babies may be ready for sleep coaching if:

- They are at least four and a half months old (adjusted age) and through the four-month sleep regression.
- Your twins' doctor has stated that it's OK for them to feed only one or two times overnight and has given you the green light to start sleep coaching.
- You are beginning to see a pattern in their sleep logs, including:
  — A regular wake time in the morning—between 6:30 and 8 AM.
  — A consistent bedtime between 6:30 and 7:30 PM.
  — One long stretch at night. (It's OK if they don't have this now, as long as they used to before the four-month regression.)

- You have a relaxing, soothing, and consistent bedtime routine.
- Your babies go down and stay down easily for naps and get the amount of sleep during the day that is expected for their age (no matter how you get them to sleep and even if they're still taking lots of short naps).
- Any feeding and health challenges (like reflux or allergies) have been either treated or are currently well managed.
- Your babies are getting enough to eat during the day (according to their age).
- Their growth is on target, and you don't need to squeeze in extra calories overnight.
- You have had some success with sleep shaping tips and either the Switcheroo or Jiggle and Soothe at bedtime.
- You and your partner are in agreement about your twins' readiness and are prepared to be a united front.
- You are prepared to stop coaching if it becomes difficult or your twins get too frustrated.
- All family members and other caregivers involved are on board.

If you feel that most of these statements describe you and your little ones, you may choose to try gentle Baby-Led Sleep Coaching.

I'd suggest you wait a few more weeks to start sleep coaching if any of the following are true for one or both of your babies:

- They still wake frequently and take full feedings at night.
- They have had a drastic change in their sleep patterns due to the four-month sleep regression, and you haven't gotten back on track yet.
- You suspect that they are still in the throes of the four-month sleep regression.
- You are not mentally ready to sleep coach (that's OK!).
- They are starting some form of childcare for the first time, and their schedule needs to change to coincide with their daycare's or nanny's schedule.
- Reflux or feeding challenges are still present.
- They have a more alert and/or sensitive temperament, and you know in your heart you need to wait and stick with sleep shaping for now.

If they are true for only one-half of your duo, you might still consider starting the sleep coaching process with the one you feel is ready.

Transitioning from Sleep Shaping to Sleep Coaching

The Baby-Led Sleep Coaching Readiness Checklist lets you know if your babies are likely to respond well to the methods we recommend in Baby-Led Sleep Coaching. As a reminder, *sleep shaping* is laying the foundation for sleep by setting up a gentle structure for the day and night; it's about the timing of sleep, following soothing routines, and creating a sleep-inducing environment. *Sleep coaching* is using strategies designed to teach your babies to fall asleep and go back to sleep *independently*—which often includes strategies that support longer stretches at night without feeding. Sleep coaching includes gently weaning a baby off sleep crutches such as pacifiers or rocking, nursing, or bottling-feeding—anything a baby needs to go to sleep and back to sleep that requires someone or something other than themselves.

All the sleep methods Kim teaches exist on a continuum that starts with the gentle foundation of Baby-Led Sleep Shaping (what you've learned so far in this book) and then move on to methods that fit under the definition of sleep coaching. But there are a few techniques that bridge the gap between the worlds of sleep shaping and sleep coaching, like the two we cover here: Jiggle and Soothe 2.0 and the Super Slow Shuffle. These build on the Jiggle and Soothe and Switcheroo you learned last month, and while we define them as sleep coaching, they share quite a bit with sleep shaping and are a gentle way to move from one to the next.

1. Jiggle and Soothe 2.0 involves waking your little ones *a bit more* than in the original Jiggle and Soothe and experimenting with patting and shushing them to sleep *a bit less*.
2. The Super Slow Shuffle involves using the basic moves from the Switcheroo to slowly change your twins' sleep associations to being put in their cribs and then patted and shushed to sleep (eventually doing the first part more quickly and patting and shushing less).

Baby-Led Sleep Shaping and Coaching ™

The gentle approach led by your duos'
unique temperaments and needs

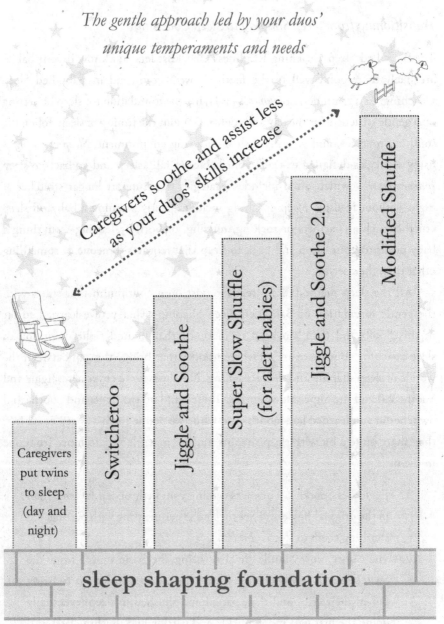

Caregivers soothe and assist less
as your duos' skills increase

Caregivers put twins to sleep (day and night)

Switcheroo

Jiggle and Soothe

Super Slow Shuffle (for alert babies)

Jiggle and Soothe 2.0

Modified Shuffle

sleep shaping foundation

Once you're confident that your twinnies have a strong sleep shaping foundation and you feel you're ready based on our readiness checklist above, you can try one of these two Gentle Sleep Coaching techniques at bedtime after a great day of naps (any way you can get them, like always!).

Sound overwhelming? Don't worry. We'll walk you through each of these in-depth.

Jiggle and Soothe 2.0 with Twins

How did your kiddos do with the Jiggle and Soothe technique from month three? After rousing them slightly, were you able to then pat and shush them back to sleep? If they responded well, try the upgraded version of this method as a next step, before moving on to the next level of sleep coaching.

1. Put each baby down to bed *already* asleep. This means that you can use whatever soothing methods you've been using (feeding, rocking, shushing, patting, etc.) to help your twinnies get there.

2. Once you lay your babies down in their crib, gently jostle them, ***waking your babies a little bit more than you did last month***. They may even look around their sleep space so they know where they are; you can talk to them and tell them where they are, as well.

3. Pat and shush your babies to get them back to sleep, just as you did last month. You can practice patting and shushing more intermittently, too! The idea is that you are doing a tiny bit less each night to put them back to sleep. You are following their lead—watching how they respond while offering reassurance as they learn, and intervening when they get too upset.

If one or both of your babies wake fully or become upset, pick them up and comfort them back to sleep. Try the steps again the next night.

You may want to make sure you have an extra pair of hands if both babies do end up waking fully and need comforting to fall back asleep (each of you can pick a "primary" baby that is your responsibility). Once you've done this a few times, if you think you can handle it solo, go for it.

The Super Slow Shuffle with Twins

The Super Slow Shuffle is an option recommended for alert babies who are past the four-month sleep regression but might not be ready for sleep coaching. We also suggest this method for parents who tell us that they, themselves, are particularly sensitive. These parents know that there will be some level of crying involved in sleep coaching but feel that it will be best for them to take the process extra slowly in hopes of reducing the crying significantly (because as a general rule, the faster a parent-baby team moves through the sleep coaching process, the more tears there are).

The Super Slow Shuffle is designed to be done with a single baby, so you'll want to either:

A. Get one baby to sleep first and then the other.
B. Do this in tandem with your partner, with each of you choosing a "primary" baby.

Here are the steps to the Super Slow Shuffle with Twins:

1. Wait to start practicing this technique at bedtime first, after a day where you were able to fill your babies' daytime sleep tanks, getting them to nap any way that you can.
2. At bedtime, follow your soothing routine like always. Make sure that this routine is consistent and well established and that bedtime is between 6:30 and 7:30 PM.
3. The first night, you'll start putting your babies to sleep the way that they are accustomed to. This might be rocking or nursing them to sleep. You're going to start by switching their association with this "going to sleep" position. For example, if you normally rock them upright to sleep on your shoulder, instead of completely putting them to sleep in that position, try slowly moving them into a more horizontal position and rocking them to sleep that way.
4. Your babies may adjust easily to this switch, or you may need to take this step slowly over several nights. There's no rush! Once they have gotten comfortable with the new position you've chosen, you can move on to the next step.

Note: These next few steps might take several nights—or your babies might adjust quickly in one night. Play it by ear!

1. With your primary baby in their new "going to sleep" position, start to—very slowly, very gently—hold them a bit farther from you, so that you have less bodily contact. You may hold them away with your arms a bit outstretched, or you might move them to your lap, keeping your arms right near them for safety. Keep them in this position until they are almost asleep.

2. Next, carry your baby *slowly* to their crib or sleep space and *very* slowly lower them in. Channel your inner ninja! Shush and speak calmly and softly as you go.

3. Keep one or both of your arms around your baby as they lay in the crib. You'll be reaching so far into the crib that it might actually feel like you are *in* it with them. (Believe it or not, we *have* had some parents get into the crib with their babies! You do not need to do this, however.)

4. Slowly remove your arm, arms, or upper body from the crib while patting and shushing your baby. You can hang over the crib and have your face close to your baby if they like it. **This is where you read your baby and follow your intuition. Really let this be a baby-led process! Some babies like a lot of close contact while others are happy with a light hand on them, just letting them know that you are still there.**

5. Slowly start to stand, continuing to pat them over the railing, as you shush them fully to sleep. (Ta-da!)

At this stage, once your babies are asleep you may decide to sleep on a mattress or chair in their room for the next several nights so you can respond quickly if they start to fuss. You have a few different options for when they wake up during the night.

- If you feel your babies are adapting well to the new method, you can repeat the Super Slow Shuffle.
- You can get them back to sleep any way you can! They are still tiny, don't forget.

Just try to make the same choice for all wakings, whether they involve a feeding or not, for the rest of the night.

Once the baby you're in charge of is comfortable with these steps, start doing less once they are in their crib and then less before putting them into the crib. Think of it like a sliding scale where you do less and less as they do more and more. If things are going well, you can try moving through the steps a bit faster to see if they have the skills to adjust to the changes at a quicker pace. You can always slow the process back down again if your kiddo isn't ready.

 Twiniversity Tip

OK, so let's just say that you've tried the Super Slow Shuffle with your twins but only one is picking it up. Reminder: This is a marathon, not a sprint, and eventually they will both get on the same page. Just stay consistent once you think you've found the right approach for each twinnie. If you feel like you need to separate them in different rooms during this process, go for it. If you feel they should stay in the same room, go for it. You are the one with your feet on the ground in *your home*.

Be Gentle with Yourself, Now and Always

A Gentle Sleep Coaching approach takes patience. Your kiddos may experience some discomfort even though you are right by their sides. If you feel that you are not up for this, it is OK to wait until you and your kiddos are both ready. You are steering this ship, so unless you feel up for the task, take a break and revisit this when you are.

Next month, if you feel your kiddos are ready, we will help you take your coaching a bit further by teaching you to put your twinnies in their cribs "calm but awake" with the Modified Shuffle.

What's the Difference Between "Drowsy but Awake" and "Calm but Awake"?

When it comes to sleep coaching, we prefer to use the phrase "calm but awake" rather than the one you might be more familiar with: "drowsy but awake." What we mean is that, rather than placing your twinnies in their crib half asleep, we want them to be awake enough to be fully aware of being placed in their crib—in other words, calm, but not drowsy.

Taking Care of You

Yes, you are sleep deprived! And this month will likely challenge you. But self-care will help you take on this challenge. It can help you stay calm and be your twinnies' detective (as always), and it prepares you for the Baby-Led Sleep Coaching in your near future. Take breaks, and if you feel you need more of them, ASK FOR THEM! It's OK. You're not a superhero. You don't have Adamantium bones (reference for all my Wolverine fans!). You are just an amazing person who did an amazing thing (having two babies at a time!) and you are doing an amazing job. Take some time to cheer yourself with a hot (or cold) cup of your favorite beverage.

Check in with Yourself (and Your Partner)

Reminder! Please make sure that you and your partner are keeping your eyes out for signs of postpartum mood disorders. See page 103 for more information and take any actions necessary to make sure both parents are getting the help they need.

Self-Care and Sleep Coaching

If you choose to sleep coach at this time, what can you do to support yourself through the process?

It might seem like you wouldn't want to add another thing to your to-do list right now—you've already got your hands full with sleep coaching! But adding self-care will help you be more patient and consistent with the coaching you're doing. As your twinnies' sleep coach, you are leading them through the process of learning to self-soothe and put themselves to sleep. How can you do that when you are run-down and dysregulated yourself?

Take a look back at some of the self-care tools we've covered and make sure you put one or two in your schedule.

What's Next?

We've taught you some next-level sleep shaping techniques, and next month we'll teach you some actual sleep coaching. I'm tearing up; I feel like we are getting close to graduation day for this phase of your twinnies' lives.

In the meantime, remember, there is always *something* you can do to support your little ones' sleep—even if your family is still navigating the four-month sleep regression.

FAST to Sleep Summary

This is going to be a doozy of a month thanks to your twins' sleep regression. Hang in there. Do what you need to do to get through, and it will (hopefully) be over before you know it. This is also the month you can start evaluating your twinnies' sleep coaching readiness. Is it time? Do you need to wait? I know you're tired, but there's no rush here. Just make sure to take care of yourself and squeeze in your naps where you can to help you get through the days ahead.

What to Focus on This Month

1. If you are *in* the four-month regression, double down on the sleep shaping elements we've taught in the first three months and implement as many as you can.

2. If you think *one or both of your twinnies* are past the four-month sleep regression and need to get back on track, add back in any sleep shaping elements that you may have let go of just to get through the regression (page 199). If you added additional feedings at night, check out page 203 for how to wean one or more of these feedings.

3. If you are back on track post-regression, review the Baby-Led Sleep Coaching Readiness Checklist (page 208) to see if you are ready for sleep coaching.

4. If your babies are back on track, try Jiggle and Soothe 2.0 (page 209) or the Super Slow Shuffle (page 210).

What Not to Worry About

Nap coaching and "keeping up with the Jones's baby"—you and your babies are on your own journey and will be ready for sleep coaching in your own time.

For a printable PDF of this month's "FAST to Sleep Summary" plus helpful book bonuses, use the QR code.

Notes

chapter seven

Your Twins' Fifth Month

Ages 16 Weeks to 20 Weeks

> *This month focuses on teaching you the elements of gentle Baby-Led Sleep Coaching for when you and your babies are ready, including how to create a successful sleep coaching plan and various methods you can incorporate into that plan. (Remember to take into consideration adjusted age, especially when it comes to sleep.)*

My Babies Aren't Newborns Anymore

Your babies have become little people with personalities of their own. And now that you have a better understanding of who they are overall, you likely have a better understanding of what works and what doesn't work for them in terms of soothing. Their development has increased their skills, and they are more capable of self-soothing. Dare we say, they might even be ready for sleep coaching!

You may still be recovering after the four-month sleep regression. If so, please don't worry! Just stick with our sleep shaping techniques until you're back on track. You can flip back to "Your Twins' Fourth Month," page 199, for all the details.

Your Developing Duo

In the fifth month, your babies are beginning to understand where objects are in relationship to other objects. They now notice that an object can be under, on, beside, or inside another object. They become more aware of the distance between themselves and you, their twin, or other caregivers. This new awareness can spark some stranger anxiety.

New abilities:

- Understanding distance and relationships between objects.
- Playing with their hands and feet.
- Grasping a toy.
- Responding to facial expressions.

Some babies can also:

- Begin to roll over in both directions.
- Mouth objects.
- Turn toward new sounds.
- Make connections between words and actions.
- Recognize their own name.
- Make vowel-consonant sounds such as *baba*.

Your babies are starting to understand object permanence. That means they're beginning to realize that even though you aren't in sight, you still exist! And that when you take their twinnie to change their diaper or grab something, you are both coming back and haven't vanished into a black hole. Object permanence hasn't fully developed, however, and they may still get a little nervous and fussy when you move out of view, as they have in the past.

They will also start to grasp the relationship between cause and effect. They can put together that if they cry, you respond, and learn to cry more deliberately to communicate. They also learn that if they drop a toy, you will pick it up for them. Parents are the best pets. We get trained really fast by our littles!

Both skills—object permanence and understanding cause and effect—can help them feel safer alone in their sleep space. They are learning that when they lie in their crib, their twin is there with them (if they are in separate cribs in the same room), and if you go to the bathroom, you still exist even if they can't see you. They have also learned to trust that when they need you and cry out, you will be there.

 Twiniversity Tip

You will probably see your kiddos interact with each other a lot more: holding hands, chewing on each other's feet, and all the other crazy wonderful things that happen when you have two babies next to each other that have literally no boundaries and often forget where they end and their twinnie starts. Have your camera ready!

Your twins' growing dexterity and ability to rake objects toward themselves with their fingers will, in a few months, turn into the *pincer grasp*: the ability to pinch one's index finger and thumb together to pick something up. This will be how they pick a pacifier up to put it back in their mouth (or their twin's mouth) when it falls out in the middle of the night. They will also soon be able to smoothly rotate their wrist to put their thumb or a few fingers in their mouth (instead of their whole fist), which some twinnies can use to self-soothe.

Stranger Anxiety

When your babies are newborns, they do not have a sense of self. Essentially, they think that the two (or three) of you are one. They smile at the feet and hands that they see waving, without realizing that they belong to them.

As your babies grow and become more aware, they gradually begin to figure out that they are their own little person with their own body, emotions, and thoughts. They finally start to understand that you, their own parent, are the one who cares for them (exciting!). When this happens, your babies may become anxious when someone new tries to hold them (even Grandma). *Stranger anxiety* is a great sign that you and your babies are bonding. Your twins know the difference between you and a stranger, and they prefer you!

We'll give you some tips for easing stranger anxiety in the following "Soothing" section.

Stranger Anxiety Versus Separation Anxiety

While they may seem similar, *stranger anxiety* and *separation anxiety* are two different things. *Stranger anxiety* may begin as early as the fifth month. Your babies can tell the difference between you and other caregivers, and they prefer you. *Separation anxiety* is when your babies get fussy and upset when they are away from you at all (no matter who else they are with). It doesn't normally begin to occur until around six or seven months and tends to come and go in waves.

Supporting Development for Better Sleep

As your twinnies continue to get used to the real world after so much time spent curled up in utero, it's important to make sure we are continuing to give their tiny bodies the chance to stretch and grow—including the opportunity to practice that holy grail of self-soothing, the ability to roll.

Tummy Time

As you know, being able to roll both ways (back to belly and belly to back) is a great self-soothing tool to add to your kiddos' baskets—and the best way to move them toward rolling, if they haven't yet mastered it, is plenty of tummy time. You can work tummy time **up to two hours total spread out throughout the day**. As always, when deciding when to have some tummy time, pick times when your babies are alert, aware, and social (but not right after feeding so they are less likely to spit up).

Teaching Rolling

Looking for motivation to make teaching your babies to roll both ways a priority? They need this skill to move them from their front to their back at night when you're not around. If they find themselves uncomfortable on their stomachs, or if you are concerned that they are not getting enough air in this position but they can only roll one direction, you'll have to regularly go in and flip them back over onto their backs.

There are several things you can do during tummy time to help your baby learn:

Rolling Front to Back

When one of your babies is on their tummy and they pull one of their legs up under them like a little frog, you can lift their same side arm and help them push off against the ground. You can then give them positive verbal feedback ("Yay!"), so they understand that they have done something awesome.

Rolling Back to Front

When one of your babies is on their back, try showing them a toy near their face or put their twin near them. You can move the toy to the floor by their side and slide it a few inches away to encourage them to reach for it, or you can move their twin a little farther away to motivate them to move in that direction. As they do, they might work hard enough to roll over on their side toward the toy or their twinnie.

For more tips on how to jazz up tummy time, see page 50.

Once your duo seems to have mastered rolling over both ways during the day, it may be time to let them be when they flip over onto their stomach at night. When they roll over in their cribs, they are just trying to get more comfortable, like you do when sleeping or napping. The American Academy of Pediatrics (AAP) supports this and considers it safe.

If one or both babies wake in the night upset after having rolled and are having some trouble getting back over, go to them and *help* them roll instead of doing it for them. Each night do less and less as they master the process on their own.

If you haven't already, you'll need to stop swaddling completely at this time. This is both for safety and to allow them to exercise their new skills and move further down the path to self-soothing.

Feeding

If you're moving to the sleep coaching phase, make sure that your twinnies are getting the recommended daily food intake for their age. That way, they won't wake up extra times at night for a snack.

Feeding at This Age

On average, babies feed *every three to four hours during the day*. There are a good number of babies this age who still wake for one feeding at night and a few who even wake for two. They will take in *between four and six ounces per feeding*.

Solids

The AAP and the World Health Organization (WHO) both recommend waiting until six months to start introducing solid foods.

Before starting to offer your twinnies solids, it is best to talk to your doctor and confirm that each baby is:

- Able to sit unassisted and has good head control (although neither is a requirement).
- Double their birth weight.
- Showing interest in what others are eating. They might even try to grab a bite from your plate!
- Taking in more than a total of 32 ounces of breast milk or formula in twenty-four hours and is fussy afterward as if they are still hungry.

Work with your pediatrician to determine if your kiddos are ready to start. This can vary and should be assessed on a case-by-case basis. If they tell you that only *one* baby is ready, it's your move on whether to start with that baby solo or wait for their twinnie to be able to get in on the action. There is no right answer here. Do what feels best to you.

Eating solids is a social and sensory experience for your twins. They get to experiment with new flavors and textures. But they may not do much actual eating at first. You'll probably see more food drip down their chins than stay in their mouths in the beginning. Learning to eat is another skill they will learn, so just be patient.

Solids and Sleep

Both *under*feeding and *over*feeding can affect sleep. As you know by now, if your babies are not getting enough to eat during the day, they will wake up more to feed at night. If your babies are getting *too much* to eat, they might wake up with tummy troubles.

I never recommend starting solids early, especially with twins and extra especially with twinnies that came on the early side. There is no need to rush this milestone unless your doc feels it might greatly benefit the twinnies for some reason. Just sit tight and wait to get the green light from your doc, and they can help you come up with an appropriate meal plan specifically for your duo.

In the meantime, please know that you *can* improve night sleep without supplementing with solids, even though other parents or consultants may tell you it is the only way. Read more about the myth about solids and sleep in "Your Twins' Fourth Month" on page 185.

Feeding Challenges in the Fifth Month

As you get ready to sleep coach or take the next step in sleep coaching, it's helpful to make sure that your babies are not experiencing any lingering feeding challenges that might affect sleep, such as reflux or GERD, reverse cycling, or new night feedings added to get through the four-month sleep regression. Take a look at the previous chapter to address these feeding challenges (though if you need more help weaning those additional feedings, we've got more for you in the "Sleep" section below). This month, we'll look at getting back on track after the four-month sleep regression and helping you if your baby goes on a feeding strike.

Getting Feeding Back on Track

If you are trying to get your babies back on track after the four-month sleep regression, we suggest looking back at your sleep log to see how long their first night stretch was before the developmental leap. If this stretch is shorter now, you'll want to work on lengthening it before you consider entering the sleep coaching phase. Please look at the suggestions for getting back on track after the four-month sleep regression in last month's "Feeding" and "Sleep" sections (pages 184 and 198).

Feeding Strikes

Feeding strikes can happen if your babies are starting daycare and, if they were exclusively breastfed, are introduced to formula and/or a bottle for the first time. Some babies will go all day without eating, waiting for their parents. This is really a thing. If this happens to you, be prepared for starving babies who eat all night to make up the calories they didn't get during the day, a.k.a. reverse cycling. If you find yourself in this situation, look at "Feeding Challenges in the Third Month" (page 157).

My Babies Started Snacking Night and Day! What Should I Do?

This is a common age for babies to start snacking a lot during the night because they have become very distracted during the day. Remember, there is a lot to see and experience, and eating can be boring by comparison.

If this happens to you, try feeding your twinnies in a quiet/boring room and using white noise if necessary to drown out all those fun sounds. You may even need to feed them more at night, temporarily, until their daytime feeding distractibility improves. If you find that only one baby is very distracted, divide and conquer if possible. You can feed one baby in one room while your partner feeds the other in another room. That way, you can focus on your distracted baby and make sure they are getting enough to eat. It's a great way to get a little one-on-one time with a kiddo, too. If you are flying solo, though, there is nothing wrong with feeding both in a less exciting area to make sure everyone is getting what they need. Do what you have to do.

Remember, however, that every baby is different! I recently worked with a family where one twin would chow down on anything put in front of them, and the other baby wanted to only breastfeed but had started snack feeding, meaning they only wanted small meals that weren't filling them up. I recommended everything I mentioned above, but we got nowhere fast. This kiddo *would not* feed. So, I made the bold suggestion that the mom do the opposite of what we had been doing: Go into a loud room that was well lit with tons of distractions. The baby was a little more attentive to feeding but still not there. Finally, we found we could get a full feed in him by walking around and feeding him at the same time. Literally. His mom was walking through the house with a baby latched on and getting some glorious feeds. The moral of the story is keep trying. Who cares if it sounds crazy as long as it works, right?

Please see "Your Twins' Third Month," page 157, for more help with distractible eaters.

 ## Attachment

As you move from Baby-Led Sleep Shaping to Baby-Led Sleep Coaching, whether that's this month or later on, you will rely on the trust you have built up and the bonds you have forged with your duo over the last several months. Keep this trust in mind as you let your babies lead you through the coaching process. Your twins still need to know that you are close by and will respond if they really need you.

 ## Soothing

By now you may feel like you have a decent handle on why your babies cry or fuss—most of the time, at least. You're finding your groove and learning to speak their language, using SOAR to help figure out their patterns and temperaments and therefore what works and what doesn't work to soothe them. On top of all that, as you have learned, your babies have more self-soothing and communication tools in their tiny toolboxes! Soothing only gets easier from here. But keep your soothing skills sharp since you'll need them down the line for sleep coaching.

Your Twins' Solidifying Self-Soothing Skills

This month your duo may exhibit even more forms of self-soothing that relate to sleep, including:

- Turning or rolling away, which they can also use at night to change positions on their own, instead of waking you to help them.
- Pushing away the bottle or breast when not hungry, which helps you understand what their night feeding needs are at this age.
- Fussing and crying and rubbing their eyes when tired, a clearer cue to help you get them to sleep before they become overtired.
- Thumb or finger sucking (more on this soon!).

These baby steps in communication will help you understand their needs even better.

Supporting Your Baby with Soothing

As your babies are starting to self-soothe, you can help them learn more techniques and remind them of their options when they are upset or fussy. This includes:

- Encouraging them to roll back over once they have rolled one direction and have gotten "stuck."
- Helping them find their thumb or fingers if you know that they find sucking particularly soothing.

Thumb-Sucking

If you're worried your kiddos' passion for thumb-sucking is going to lead to hefty braces bills later down the line, you can take a deep breath. Pediatric dentists have confirmed that a child's need for orthodontic care is more related to their genetics than chewing on their little paws.

Thumb-sucking has a lot of negative connotations, but I'll tell ya, there are pretty sweet benefits, too. As you know, thumb-sucking (or the "hand sandwich," where they put their entire hand in their mouth) allows a baby to self-soothe at a young age. And if your baby is sucking their thumb, it may mean that something in their world (external environment or even inside them) has made them uncomfortable. Thumb-sucking can become a clue to their needs. It may be a sign that they are getting tired and ready for sleep. Or it may be a sign of anxiety, showing they need some help getting regulated as they try to process and understand a new environment or new people.

You may not be able to control if your baby becomes a thumb-sucker; you might have even seen one or both of your babies sucking on their thumbs in utero! Don't let it bother you too much. Many kiddos outgrow it as they build more self-soothing skills. I'll tell you this, too: Don't be too shocked if one twinnie ends up sucking on the other twinnie's thumb. My twins often chewed and sucked on their twin's hand more than they did their own. Yeah, those two had no personal space. I often felt that they didn't know where they ended and where their twin began. Moments like that make me realize how lucky I am to have twins and how boring it must be to have only a singleton.

Soothing Challenges in the Fifth Month

Although your babies have some new self-soothing options this month, you are still their primary source of regulation, and your help is still very much needed when it comes to getting their needs met. And as you saw in the "Development" section, the biggest new challenge they may be experiencing this month is stranger anxiety.

Soothing Stranger Anxiety

Remember, stranger anxiety is actually a good sign! It means that your babies are creating a strong bond with you. It can still be difficult to handle, though.

Here are a few things that you can do to help your twinnies become comfortable with new visitors and caregivers:

- Be friendly. Your babies are learning social cues from you, so make sure to demonstrate how much you like and trust this new person before you hand them over.
- Don't stress. If your babies have a meltdown while someone else is holding them, don't get upset. Just calmly take them back into your arms to soothe them.

- Respond to them with comfort and empathy. Offer soothing objects, like a pacifier or a lovey.
- If they are soothed by sucking their thumb or fingers, encourage them to do so by bringing their hand to their mouth. You may see that they naturally start to suck their thumb on their own.
- Take extra time. The first time you leave your babies with a new caregiver, take a few extra minutes to play with them *and* the new caregiver. This is another way of showing them this new person can be trusted.
- Always say goodbye. Create a routine for before you leave (and one for your return!). Your babies will start to recognize these transitions and anticipate what comes next.
- Don't linger. After saying goodbye, leave quickly to avoid triggering a meltdown.
- Keep trying. It may take your twins a while to adjust to a new person or new environment. You just have to be persistent.

In the meantime, you may want to inform family and friends who want to come and see the sideshow that is your new life with twins what to expect and not take it personally!

Eventually your duo will get over their anxiety around strangers. Stay connected and close during their peak anxiety time, and do the best you can to make them feel safe, secure, and loved.

Stranger Danger

I feel like I have to say this for any new parents in the room who feel like they need permission to trust their instincts: If someone wants to hold your kiddos that you don't like or trust, *don't hand them over.* Just because someone is visiting doesn't mean they have a right to hold your kiddos. Yes, even if they brought a gift. Be polite, but don't ever feel pressured to do anything that makes you feel uncomfortable. If someone is visiting that you know you're not a big fan of, tell your partner ahead of time so they can cover for you if necessary. Heck, go hide in a room and tell them you have to breastfeed—even if you're the dad! Just please, don't put yourself into any uncomfortable positions. Period. The end. You have enough to worry about—don't add anything else to your list.

 ## Temperament

We are finally at the age when experts all agree that your babies' temperaments are truly emerging. You may have learned that one or both of your babies were alert several months ago, but now you're recognizing the nuances of the traits specifically associated with alert babies. Maybe one of your kiddos is particularly sensitive but not intense. They may get fussy more quickly in a loud room, but their fussiness isn't any more intense than that of other babies. Or maybe they both go from zero to sixty in three seconds flat when they get hungry, but one of your twins hates a dirty diaper, and the other doesn't.

Nurturing Your Babies' Unique Natures

Over the years both scientists and parents have wondered about how much we are able to mold a baby's temperament. Research now suggests that 50 percent of temperament is based on nature and 50 percent is based on nurture. When it comes to sleep, we find that *more* of a baby's temperament is based on nature. We regularly hear the myth that parents can train their babies to sleep in loud environments. Unfortunately, this isn't true. Either your babies' temperaments will allow them to do so (if you are lucky!) or they won't.

You've learned that attachment comes from being properly attuned to your babies and their particular needs. Learning their temperaments—their natures—allows you to nurture them as they are instead of trying to fit a square peg into a round hole. Our aim is not to change our kiddos but rather to accept who we have been given . . . even (especially!) if their temperaments are not what we envisioned or wanted. You'll continue to learn to love your time with your babies even when they are not who you imagined they'd be. Give your babies the chance to be who they are. You will be rewarded greatly, and so will they!

Sleep Coaching Alert Babies

You can expect your alert baby or babies to push back against sleep shaping and sleep coaching. When you change familiar patterns, these smart little cookies will let you know that they notice. They will also let you know, loud and clear, that they don't like it. Do what you can to push through. As long as you are present and supportive, it's OK for them to hate the change. If you can acknowledge their difficulty and just keep going, they will use their powerful brain to pick up on the new pattern—and alert babies love a good pattern.

The worst thing you can do with an alert baby is to try and try a new approach—and then just give up and do whatever works. When your babies' sleep and temperaments meet, sleep has to win. If you're inconsistent, your children won't overlook it. If you start out patting and shushing and then end up feeding them to sleep, for example, they will know that feeding is "on the table" as a possibility, and they just have to find it. The next time you try to hold out, it can be ten times harder. Set your mind to whatever you are choosing to do and try not to waffle. Remember, you have to stay one step ahead of your alert child(ren). They don't miss a thing!

Parents of Alert Babies Are the Ones That Seek the Most Help

Over the years, around 75 percent of the clients who have sought help from Kim have had alert babies—because alert babies often have sleep difficulties. They have a harder time shutting the world out to go to sleep, and so they often need ALL of the sleep environment recommendations: a clear pre-sleep routine (which sometimes needs to be longer), quiet, room-darkening shades, consistent sleep times, and sleeping in their own sleep space. They are not as adaptable for the first few years and won't easily sleep in the car or in a stroller (or on vacation!).

If you've been blessed with an amazing active, engaged, tenacious child, you also might be particularly sleep deprived. Please don't be upset if you've gotten to this point and your alert baby is still not sleeping well. You may have to implement

Kim's Baby-Led Sleep Shaping and Sleep Coaching elements at a slower pace, but there is sleep at the end of the tunnel!

To get one-on-one assistance from a personal twin-specific sleep coach, use the QR code.

Getting You and Your Babies to Sleep

In their fifth month, your twins may be sleeping much longer stretches at night, or even be sleeping through the night, which is defined as sleeping six hours or more in a stretch. Yes, you just read that right. Six hours or more in a stretch is considered "sleeping through the night." Did you think your babies were going to sleep a solid ten hours or so? That will come later. For now, their tiny little bellies still hit "empty" sooner than you may like. But for most parents, even six solid hours can feel like you've won the lotto.

While some babies may be getting some solid shut-eye, a good number of babies this age still wake for one feeding at night, and a few even wake for two. Remember, it's always important to speak to your doctor about when you can officially drop overnight feeds. Don't go rogue and just start dropping bottles or boob time. Make sure everything is on track, especially if your duo was born on the early side.

Sleep Needs in Healthy Full-Term Babies

The typical sleep average for your babies in this fifth month is ***ten to twelve hours of sleep per night and three and a half to four hours during the day spread out over three to four naps.*** Your baby should also be able to stay awake anywhere from two to two and a quarter hours between naps, depending on nap length.

Ready for Sleep Coaching?

Not all babies are ready for sleep coaching at this stage. Kim has worked with babies as old as eight and nine months who just weren't yet ready. Sometimes the reason has to do with a baby's temperament, or with a difficult beginning, prematurity, or an illness that they are getting over. We need to take all these things into account when creating a plan and choosing a start date.

If you are wondering if your twins might be ready for sleep coaching, please take a look at the Baby-Led Sleep Coaching Readiness Checklist on page 205– 206.

As you prepare to begin sleep coaching, put that detective hat on again! Make sure you're taking into account any lingering issues that might affect the success of your plan. Was there a particularly traumatic birth that still requires some recovery for either you or your twins? Are you or your partner feeling guilty about returning to full-time work? Have there been feeding difficulties or any underlying medical concerns? If you answer yes to any of these questions, sleep coaching might be a bit more challenging for your family, and you may want to press pause and revisit this page in a week or so. Slow and steady wins the race, as they say.

I want you to commit to only what *you* feel comfortable with and can follow through with consistently. Go over your goals and look at your family's schedule. Do you feel like you are particularly sleep deprived and need to address your twins' sleep sooner rather than later? Do you have the recommended three weeks to devote to the process? Or would you feel better waiting if you're not feeling in a rush?

In the rest of this section, we'll introduce you to some Gentle Sleep Coaching techniques for both bedtime and nap time, and then help you create your personalized Baby-Led Sleep Coaching plan.

Are We There Yet?

If you don't feel like your twins (or you!) are quite ready for sleep coaching, revisit the sleep shaping sections in "Your Twins' Third Month" and "Your Twins' Fourth Month" (pages 167 and 199). Remember, there is no rush here. Yes, you're tired, but we have to make sure the babies (and you) are ready before we move to the next step.

If you are feeling great about their sleep shaping foundation and you're still ready to keep moving forward on their sleep adventure, even if you aren't ready for the Gentle Sleep Coaching described in this chapter, you can try Jiggle and Soothe 2.0 (page 209) or the Super Slow Shuffle (page 210) as an interim step.

How Fast "Should" I Sleep Coach?

How quickly you choose to sleep coach will depend on your goals for your twins' sleep (and your own). It will also depend on their temperaments—and yours. As you know, the sleep coaching that we recommend is gentle, but changing patterns almost always results in a few tears. And not just theirs—you may even shed a few of your own. We find that when parents speed up the process, the tears tend to increase a bit. **If you are particularly sensitive to your kiddos' cries, you might want to go slow.**

With alert babies, going too fast can be an issue—but so can going too slow because they might get too comfortable at one stage of the process, making it more difficult to move them to the next. You'll need to find a nice middle ground, keep evaluating how they are doing at your chosen speed, and adjust as needed.

To be clear, it's OK to go VERY slowly if you find that's what is best for your duo. Alert babies often need microsteps in the sleep coaching process. You may feel frustrated that they can't move faster. And you may feel like you are the only one moving as slow as a turtle. But trust me, other parents of alert babies are right there with you!

Your Sleep Log Will Keep You Sane

Remember to keep sleep and feeding logs during your sleep coaching adventures, so you can see any patterns, good or bad, as they start to emerge and assess what is working and what is not. It is too difficult to keep all the information you want to remember in your head for two babies; the nights in particular will blur together. It will be difficult to see progress . . . and you don't want to miss that!

We recommend recording the following:

- What time you put your babies down for the night.
- How long it took them to get to sleep.
- What your babies did—for example, fuss, cry, roll over, any other soothing behaviors.
- How much and how long they cried.

- What you did or didn't do—for example, patting, shushing, picking them up to calm them.
- How often your babies woke, what you did at each waking, and how long they were awake.
- The number of night feedings.
- What time you started the day.

You'll also want to log all nap times and lengths and daytime feedings. If you need to figure out a sleep coaching challenge later, you can look back to see if the cause might be a change in their behavior or activities.

Don't forget, you can do this all on the Twiniversity app.

Skip Sleep Coaching While Away

No matter how desperate you get, start your sleep coaching adventure in your own home. I've seen folks traveling to see family and think, *I have more help here, let me start sleep coaching so I'll have more support*. Traveling is hard enough with twinnies, and throwing in an epic event like sleep coaching while away from home is a challenge I'd like you to take a pass on. You'll have an easier time logistically and emotionally with the creature comforts of your own home around you. And you're not the only one that will have an easier time—the twins will, too.

Baby-Led Sleep Coaching for Twins

When you commit to sleep coaching, you're committing to teaching your twins to learn to fall asleep without your help. Kim and I want you to provide them with support while remembering that sleep is a learned skill—one that they learn with your support and guidance.

Kim's sleep coaching method for twins this age who are developmentally ready is called the Modified Shuffle.

Introducing the Modified Shuffle (It's Not the Same as the "Regular"
Sleep Lady Shuffle)

When I met Kim many years ago, her main method of sleep coaching was called
"the Sleep Lady Shuffle." Easy to remember, since she *is* The Sleep Lady. That
method is taught at length in her book *The Sleep Lady's Good Night, Sleep Tight*,
and it's designed to help children from six months to six years old. The Modified
Shuffle is for kiddos under six months. It includes many of the same steps as the
Sleep Lady Shuffle but goes at a slower pace.

Here, we've customized the Modified Shuffle specifically for twin families,
since it's much easier if you have more than one adult available. (If you need to do
this 100 percent solo, it's not ideal, but it's also not impossible. We'll outline the
steps below.)

I can't wait to tell you all about it. Let's jump in!

The Modified Shuffle, Step-by-Step—for Twins

The step-by-step process of the Modified Shuffle allows you to gradually diminish
your role in helping your twins fall asleep, giving them the room to figure out how
to soothe themselves. The idea is to be their coach, not their crutch.

Think of the Modified Shuffle as a kind of weaning for sleep: You are there
providing physical and verbal reassurance while, over the course of a week or two,
doing less and less as your babies learn the skill of putting themselves to sleep
independently.

 Twiniversity Tip

You may want to split up your twins temporarily if one twin is ready for coaching
and the other isn't. While you're in the process of coaching the baby who's ready,
consider moving their twinnie into a different room so you can focus all your attention on the first baby. However, if you feel both of your kiddos are ready to start the

Modified Shuffle, then keep them in the same room. Yes, they will wake each other up, but you and a buddy will tag team and coach them each back to sleep. Plus, twins are amazing at learning to sleep through each other's crying!

Getting Started with the Modified Shuffle with Your Twins

After a great day of naps (any way you can get them), go through your standard bedtime routine (e.g., diaper change, pajamas on, into sleep sack, feeding). After the last step of this soothing routine, turn off the lights and turn on your dim night-light (this low light will allow you to safely navigate your twins' room for sleep coaching).

Place your babies in their sleep space "calm but awake." This means that you have not put them to sleep with any assistance like nursing, rocking, walking, or patting, but they are dry, fed, warm enough, loved, and starting to get tired when you put them in their cribs.

Nights 1–3

For these first three nights, we recommend having your partner or a buddy at your side. You can each pick a baby to dedicate yourself to and focus all your energy on. This will help you build confidence, since you won't feel like you need to split yourself in two. If you are flying solo, take a deep breath and do the best you can.

Stay close to your baby or babies by sitting or standing next to the crib and comfort them *with touch and verbal reassurance* until they fall asleep. You can pat, gently rock back and forth, jiggle, shush, and provide verbal reassurance. Whatever works for you and your babies.

Using touch, eye contact, and/or your voice, calm them down as needed. These first few nights are when they might need some extra soothing, which is why we recommend you don't fly solo unless necessary. *Yes, you can pick them up*—but once they're calm, put them back in their cribs.

Some babies don't like a lot of patting but may be comforted by shushing. If you feel they are looking at you too much, sit on the floor and try comforting them through the slats of the crib (versus over the top of the rail) and continuing the shushing and vocal calming to see if that works. You may find that your babies seem more upset when you make eye contact. If so, that's an easy fix—just close your eyes!

If space permits—and especially if you're doing this solo—consider standing or sitting between your babies' cribs so that you can easily reach both of them. Your body will block your twinnies from seeing each other—something that may give each of them a boost of eye contact–fueled adrenaline. Think about it—when you had a sleepover with your bestie, and you rolled over and were face-to-face, you'd end up chatting more versus going to sleep. Yeah, your twinnies are the BFFs in the situation. Just replace "chatting" with "crying."

The goal is to help your twins fall asleep *in their cribs*—even if that means your entire upper body is in the crib with them (assuming that seems to help, of course!). Experiment with what works for you and your babies.

Don't worry about doing too much patting and shushing the first night, but it's essential that each night you gradually reduce your physical reassurance and use more verbal reassurance. And know that it's OK to practice these steps for a few nights longer if you have a particularly sensitive baby (just as we suggested with the Super Slow Shuffle).

Nights 4–6

You did it! Welcome to phase two. While you and your partner/buddy may have made one heck of a tag team for the last few nights, it's time to make this a solo act. If you've been flying solo, you're already golden.

Put your babies in their cribs and sit a few feet away, continuing to offer verbal reassurance—for example, shushing or singing intermittently.

If your babies are particularly fussy, first wait a beat, but then you can come back to the side of the crib to verbally soothe them. If shushing and the sound of your voice doesn't soothe them, you can go back to patting them. But you'll be doing less patting going forward, and therefore this step will be more difficult if you were using a lot of touch during the first three nights.

A particularly upset baby may need more than patting to calm down. They may need to be picked up. But once they are calm, you'll want to put them back in their crib and see how little verbal or physical reassurance you can give them before they are calm enough for you to move back to where you were sitting.

Nights 7–9

You are doing great and you've come a long way. Kim and I are very proud of you. YAY!

Each night, move your chair incrementally farther away from their cribs, toward the door, until you no longer feel they need you to stay in the room—because finally, they are easily going to sleep on their own.

 Twiniversity Tip

When working as a team sleep coaching your duo, you may want to make it a tag team! You can switch who is soothing which baby as often as you feel comfortable or not at all. It's up to you how you want to do this; just communicate clearly with your partner so each of you know your role for each coaching session and what to expect from each other during that time.

Guidelines for the Modified Shuffle (Hint: Bookmark This Page!)

These are your rules of engagement for standing and sitting by your twins' cribs as you do the Modified Shuffle.

- You can **stroke, shush, pat, and rub your babies—but not constantly.** The idea is to do this intermittently so that these actions don't become a new sleep association. You don't want your little ones to expect you to pat and shush them to sleep every night. (While we did practice this in sleep shaping, we have moved on to sleep coaching now.)
- You'll want to **carefully manage your level of touch**—again, to avoid creating a new sleep association. In other words, don't let your children fall asleep holding your finger, or they'll expect to do this each time they need to get back to sleep. Plus, when you move, they're likely to wake and you'll have to start again.
- As you move away from your twins' cribs, **reduce the amount or volume of verbal reassurance** so that your babies can learn to sleep without it.
- You can pick up your babies and soothe them if they become too distraught to fall asleep on their own, but **try not to hold them too long and definitely not to sleep.** Always try some variation of shushing or patting first to see if that calms them.
- Throughout the last several months you have become your twins' expert. **Use your intuition and past experience** to gauge how much frustration they can handle with you by their side.
- **It's OK to move at a slower pace** than outlined here. You can spend two extra nights patting them through the bars of their cribs. Or you can spend an extra night staying by their cribs if you think they need it. You can spend more time on any step at any point if you feel your twins aren't ready to move to the next one. And if you feel like one of your kiddos isn't ready but the other is, you can coach them one at a time. See our "Twiniversity Tip" on page 238.

What If My Babies Cry?

There is no way to get your twinnies to have a cryless experience while learning the skill of soothing themselves. Babies cry. It's how they communicate. They're good at it. So, yeah, they are going to cry a little bit.

Remember, if you're worried about one baby's crying waking their twin, don't. Most of the time, a twin's crying is like white noise to their sibling. They hear it, but they don't do much about it.

In general, a parent's goal is to have as few tears touch their babies' sweet little cheeks as possible. Right? But remember, while using a gentler sleep coaching method will definitely reduce crying, that does not mean your baby will not cry *at all*. They are learning a new skill! And the amount and intensity of that crying will depend on temperament, past experience, age, and more.

I really do *know* how hard it is to listen to your babies cry. And yes, when you have twins, they do cry in surround sound. Listening to my twins cry broke my heart into a million little pieces. I always reminded myself of two things: (1) if they are crying, they are breathing; and (2) a little crying here and there didn't make me a bad parent because crying is what babies do. For those little ones that are nonverbal, crying is how they let us know they are uncomfortable or frustrated, or that they need to be moved into a different position. **Sleep coaching is all about letting your babies sit with a little frustration while you provide support so that they can successfully learn to sleep on their own.**

The sleep coaching process can be a little stressful for everyone involved. Sometimes, babies are simply picking up on *your* reaction to this new way of going to sleep. If you suspect your twins are getting stressed because *you're* feeling anxious, don't leave the room. Instead, just back off a bit, or test sitting on the floor next to the crib and using only your voice to see if that helps. It may be that a calmer you is just what they were craving. If you are feeling anxious, having a different caregiver handle the coaching process might also be a good option.

 Twiniversity Tip

If you go in with a defeatist attitude about sleep coaching, you will be defeated. Stay positive and take each moment as it comes. You CAN handle everything that is thrown at you, and if you feel you can't or that this process is a waste of time and overwhelming you, hit pause and wait till you're ready. You WILL get this. Your twins WILL sleep. YOU need to be ready, not just them.

Prolonged, unsupported crying is harmful for babies, so we don't want you to leave your twins to cry unsupported. We want you to be right there reassuring them. Even so, you may be wondering: What's *too much* crying? How long is too long? You are the best person to determine this, not us. You know your babies best! However, if your babies have not had any calm periods in the last ten to fifteen minutes, then please pick them up to calm them. It's OK. You aren't ruining them. A baby who cries (even on and off) for any longer can end up too upset to learn anything new—so help that little puppy out.

If you decide you are not comfortable with the crying and are beginning to question whether your twins are ready for sleep coaching, it is fine to stop and wait to start again when they are older—it will never be too late to sleep coach. The same goes for if you realize that your babies are particularly sensitive. And if you'd like to continue with sleep coaching but would like an even slower version, we suggest the Super Slow Shuffle in "Your Twins' Fourth Month" (page 210).

Baby-Led Sleep Coaching—It's Time!

OK gang, we've broken Baby-Led Sleep Coaching into three phases:

- Coaching at bedtime only (**Phase 1: At Bedtime Only**, page 242).
- Coaching both at bedtime and during night wakings (**Phase 2: Addressing Nighttime Wakings and Feedings**, page 246).
- Coaching at bedtime, during night wakings, and for naps (**Phase 3: Nap Coaching**, page 252).

Please choose the starting place that is the best match for your twinnies' temperaments and your own. Some parents may decide to skip ahead to coaching their twinnies both at bedtime and back to sleep when they wake at night. Some may even decide to sleep coach their kiddos from the beginning at all three times: at bedtime, during the night, and for naps. Always start coaching your babies at bedtime (Phase 1) after a great day of naps any way you can get them (and yes, it's OK to use all your sleep crutches for those naps!).

Phase 1: At Bedtime Only

They slept great all day, right? OK. Just checking. (I sound like a broken record, I know.)

During Phase 1:

- Bedtime: Sleep coach following the Modified Shuffle.
- Night wakings with feeding: Put your baby (or babies) back to sleep using your usual method (often this is nursing or bottle-feeding them until they are asleep before gently transferring them to their crib).
- Night wakings with no feeding: Put your baby (or babies) back to sleep using your usual method (for example, feeding, rocking, or holding to sleep before gently transferring them to their crib).
- Nap time: Put your baby (or babies) to sleep using your usual method before gently transferring them to their crib.

Note that you may find that your usual methods stop working during night wakings. If so, you may have to start sleep coaching back to sleep during night wakings as well; see Phase 2: Addressing Nighttime Wakings and Feedings.

How to Start the Modified Shuffle If Your Babies Are Fed to Sleep

Many babies feed to sleep (and then again back to sleep), but the purpose of Baby-Led Sleep Coaching is to help them learn how to get to sleep without being nursed or bottle-fed. In order to switch their association away from feeding to sleep:

- Start the night with your standard soothing bedtime routine.
- Feed them with the light on, both so that they stop associating feeding with falling asleep in the dark and so that you can watch to see when they are done feeding and are about to fall asleep.
- Before they do, unlatch them or remove the bottle and gently put them in their crib "calm but awake."
- Now start the steps to the Modified Shuffle.

Feeding *back* to sleep is such a common sleep crutch that we've devoted an entire phase of Baby-Led Sleep Coaching to it. Please refer to Phase 2 (page 246) for how to handle night wakings.

How to Start the Modified Shuffle If Your Babies Are Rocked, Held, or Walked to Sleep

Babies who are accustomed to bouncing or swinging to sleep will particularly miss this movement and activity when you start sleep coaching. If you haven't yet, please go back and read the recommendations for the Modified Shuffle on page 235 regarding having a buddy help ya—it's particularly helpful here!

- Before starting your pre-bed routine, each person should walk one baby around the bedroom or rock them in the bedroom (with the light on) to create a positive association between the room and sleep as a precursor to sleep coaching. After this soothing, go ahead and run through their standard pre-bed routine. Sometimes folks do some rocking and swaying again as they turn off the light and put their twinnie in the crib.
- As you lay your twinnie in their crib "calm but awake," lean over into the crib and continue rocking or bouncing as you very slowly put your baby down. This will give them more of the movement they're used to as they get settled in. Experiment with what works for you and each baby. There is no one way to do this! And each of your babies may need something differ-ent. Remember, you are the one who calls the shots, since Kim and I can't be next to you in anything other than spirit until teleportation is invented.
- Follow recommendations for the Modified Shuffle, being very conserva-tive with the "pick up to calm" suggestions. Sometimes babies whose sleep crutch has been holding or rocking will fall asleep in your arms in a min-ute or two when they are picked up to be calmed—which can train them to cry (something we want to avoid!).

If these steps sound like too much all at once, you can follow the steps to the Super Slow Shuffle in "Your Twins' Fourth Month" (page 210). It takes your babies through the process at an even slower rate that might work to help them switch their sleep associations.

Your Nap Plan While Sleep Coaching at Bedtime Only

If you choose to start with only Phase 1, you will create a sleep plan later in this chapter that includes sleep coaching only at bedtime. The nap section of your plan will be to get naps "any way you can get them" while you focus on bedtime, until you feel that your babies can be put down in their cribs for bed with minimal patting and shushing.

If your babies nap well during the day, they will sleep better at night. This is because it is more difficult for them to fall asleep and stay asleep when they get into an overtired state. So, while you are not yet sleep coaching your duo during naps, you still want to pay attention to them to make sure they are getting enough sleep.

Fortunately, changes to their circadian rhythms at this age makes this easier! You are probably starting to notice your twins' naps take on a more consistent schedule. You may have already started to see signs that their morning nap now happens at the same time every day.

NAP EXPECTATIONS

Let's take a look at what typical infant naps look like right now:

- Your babies should be napping **at least three to four times a day for at least forty-five minutes at a time** (if their naps are shorter—which sometimes happens during sleep coaching—they may need five naps a day). You are working toward **a total of three and a half to four hours of daytime sleep**.
- Naps average between forty-five minutes and two and a half hours.
- Most babies do not transition from three to four naps down to two to three naps until six to eight months. They then transition to two naps after around nine months if they are sleeping well at night.

It's not uncommon for some babies this age to take several forty-five-minute naps and then slowly, and on their own, shift to two longer naps and a third shorter nap (which is common for six- to eight-month-olds).

Because nap lengths still vary at this age, this can, of course, affect their wake windows (how long they are typically able to stay awake between naps without getting fussy):

- Shorter nap (forty-five minutes to one hour) = shorter wake window (sixty to ninety minutes)
- Longer nap (one hour or longer) = longer wake window (ninety minutes to two and a half hours)

When you look at your sleep and feeding logs, you'll get a sense of their usual wake windows. You'll probably notice that their first nap of the day typically comes after a shorter wake window than usual.

In order to fill your twinnies' nap tanks during sleep coaching, your goal is to get them three and a half to four hours of naps a day. This is a range, and the total amount depends both on how much sleep you feel each twinnie needs to be well rested in a twenty-four-hour period and on how they are sleeping at night. If they are waking more at night, they will be extra tired in the morning, so be ready for their first nap to fall a bit earlier and for them to require more sleep during the day. The number of naps they need will depend on the length of each nap.

For example, if one of your babies takes only forty-five-minute naps, then they will likely need more naps per day than their twin who naps for an hour or longer each time. Do what you have to, to fill as much of their sleep tanks as you can. If you have to walk around the block wearing one and strolling with the other to get them to sleep, go for it.

Here are our recommendations for getting good daytime sleep:

- Find the time that your babies often wake in the morning, then regulate their wake-ups at that time going forward (an irregular wake-up confuses their internal clock). If one is an early riser and one wakes a little later, try to make their regular wake-up time somewhere in the middle.
- Hold off their first nap until after 8 AM to encourage an appropriate wake time.
- If they nap before then, you'll usually find that they end up with an early rising problem.
- For the rest of your twins' naps, watch for sleepy cues and keep an eye on their wake windows. (Staying awake longer than two and a half hours can make it more difficult for them to fall asleep, cause restless sleep, and lead to difficulty staying asleep.)

- Provide an ideal daytime sleep environment (page 92).
- Commit to a pre-nap routine (your standard daytime pre-sleep routine).

 Twiniversity Tip

If you find that your babies have different sleep needs (more common with fraternal twins), try not to let their schedules get too off-kilter from each other. When possible, try to keep the variation in their sleeping and eating schedules to a difference of no more than thirty minutes.

GENTLE NAP EXTENSION STRATEGIES

If one or both of your babies regularly take short naps and still seem tired when they wake up, you can try to extend their naps by going into their sleep space five minutes before their usual wake-up time and, when they start to rouse a little, soothing them back to sleep, whether by patting them or picking them up to rock them back to sleep. This will help them connect their nap cycles, rather than waking fully between them.

Keep in mind that the last nap of the day is usually the shortest—often just forty-five minutes—you want your babies to wake from their last nap two hours before bedtime. So, you may not want to extend this one!

Phase 2: Addressing Nighttime Wakings and Feedings

Once your babies have gotten used to going to sleep in their cribs with minimal support (very little shushing or patting), it's time to move on to coaching when your babies wake throughout the night.

When Your Babies Wake Frequently and Need Help to Go Back to Sleep

First, you'll want to focus on sleep coaching when your babies wake in the night and they don't need to nurse or take a bottle. You and your pediatrician may have figured out that even though they are waking up frequently, they don't need a feed each time, or even at all. They are just not yet able to put themselves back to sleep without you rocking/holding/walking them. If this is the case with your duo, you can plan to treat every night waking the same: Follow the Modified Shuffle to get them back to sleep each time until 6 AM.

Remember, if you're sleep coaching this solo, have backup in case you need it. Always tend to the baby that you think is under the most stress first. Try to have their cribs close enough together that you can lay a hand on each of them at the same time. If you need to pick one up, do so, calm them, and put them down, and then repeat with the other one.

When Your Babies Wake Frequently to Feed: Weaning Night Feedings

If your twins are waking frequently at night because they got used to eating at those times, a big part of your sleep coaching plan will involve weaning them off many of these night feedings.

We recommend reviewing your babies' gestational age, health, and feeding patterns with your doctor to determine whether they need those extra meals/snacks during the night. If your doctor says that your twins need to eat overnight, ask them how many feedings they recommend. You can then gently wean your duo off the feedings that are no longer necessary.

It's important to determine whether your twins are getting enough calories throughout the day. Since many babies do wake up in the night because they are hungry and need to eat (especially in the first six months), it may be possible to shift some of their calorie intake to the daytime. This on its own can theoretically reduce night wakings and therefore improve night sleep.

Please keep in mind that if your twinnies are used to eating in the night, it doesn't matter whether they are actually hungry or the night feedings are just a habit—it will still *feel* like hunger. Therefore, we always recommend a gentle/gradual approach to night weaning.

HOW TO GENTLY REDUCE NIGHT FEEDS

Remember, it is perfectly normal for your five-month-old twins to have at least one feeding during the night. Most parents at this age cut the number of night feedings rather than eliminate them all together. (If you want to wean night feedings entirely, see "When Your Babies No Longer Need to Feed at Night," page 250.)

If you are reducing to one feeding, pick the feeding that you want to *keep* for the night (we recommend choosing the one where they currently chow down the best). At that feeding, let them feed as much and as long as necessary. Once they are done eating, coach them back to sleep if needed.

For other wakings, you have two options:

Option 1 is to coach your twins back to sleep with no feeding for all their wakings before 6 AM.

Option 2 is to feed them at their other wakings, but slowly, over the course of three or four nights, reduce the ounces or minutes they are fed (except at the one feeding time you chose to keep) until, eventually, you're not feeding them at all but rather coaching them back to sleep if they continue to wake. This is the more gradual approach. You'll remain cribside practicing the steps of the Modified Shuffle for each nonfeed waking. *Note*: If you try option 2 and they start to cry because they are too awake after their feeding, then you will be better off stopping this approach the next night and instead coaching them back to sleep for all wakings *other* than the one you wish to keep.

While you reduce night feeds, be prepared to feed your baby more frequently during the day.

Some sleep experts suggest pushing a baby's feed later and later each night in order to slowly lengthen their sleep stretches. We don't recommend this; we find that this type of approach leaves parents exhausted, which makes sleep coaching more difficult because tired parents end up being more inconsistent. The only time we've seen this work is with night nannies or newborn care specialists who are in the home solely for the purpose of supporting the baby during the nighttime hours.

Now let's talk about the one feeding that you plan to keep. There are two methods to try: dream feeds and set-time feeds.

Dream Feeds

With a dream feed, you are feeding your babies before they wake and cry in an attempt to extend the length of the sleep stretch that follows. (For more on dream feeds, flip back to page 138.) You can use dream feeds in conjunction with reducing ounces over the course of a few nights as well. To do this, schedule one dream feed (offering the full amount of milk) and then reduce the ounces in the other feedings over the course of a few nights.

Set-Time Feeds

Some babies do not respond well to dream feeds and will not feed well, only to wake shortly afterward. If this sounds like one or both of your babies, try a set-time feed instead. With set-time feeds, you choose the time at which to feed them at night (for example, at the first waking after 10 PM or the first waking after 2 AM). For any other night wakings, you coach your twins back to sleep without a feed.

So, for example, if your set-time feed is the first waking after 2 AM and your twins wake up at 1 AM, you wouldn't let them cry until 2 AM and then feed them. You'd coach them back to sleep at 1 AM and then feed them the next time they wake after 2 AM.

When the goal is to move from multiple feedings down to only one feeding, look at your logs to see which of the night feedings is when they take in most of their nutrition. For example, you may find that the 1 AM feed is the biggest, in which case your set-time feeding should be the first waking after midnight. When your babies wake up for the first time after midnight, you will feed them and put them back to bed.

It's OK if you need to reassure your babies back to sleep after their dream feed or set-time feed or if they fall asleep as they're finishing. For all other wakings, you will coach your twins back to sleep.

If you are breastfeeding, consider having another caregiver or the other parent coach your twinnies back to sleep at nonfeeding times, as it might be easier for your babies—they won't be expecting that person to nurse them.

When Your Babies No Longer Need to Feed at Night: Weaning All Night Feedings

You and your pediatrician may decide that you can wean your twins off night feedings altogether. If you have already weaned them off all feedings but one, and now want to wean them off their remaining feeding, try the Four-Night Phase Out:

- Whether breastfeeding or bottle-feeding, feed your babies just once during the night for three nights, using a set-time or dream feed. Reduce the feeding amount at this last feeding over the course of these three nights as described on page 203. Then don't feed them again until 6 AM. If they wake up other times, offer physical and verbal assurance to coach them back to sleep.
- On the fourth night, drop the feeding entirely and comfort them back to sleep each time they wake. Use the guidelines for the Modified Shuffle to soothe them, and only pick them up to calm them if they get overly upset.

Saying Goodbye to Mr. Pacifier

 Most pediatricians recommend weaning your kids off the pacifier by eighteen months to two years, but if your babies are waking up a lot at night seeking their bobo (as it was called in my house) and they don't know how to replug it themselves yet, you might want to tackle pacifier weaning now. Be prepared for a few nights of sheer terror. OK, I'm being dramatic. It won't be fun, but you can totally do it.

As with most of our sleep-related coaching, you'll want to start at bedtime after a great day of naps. You'll put your babies down in their cribs after their standard soothing pre-bed routine without their pacifier. Then follow the steps for the Modified Shuffle.

Knowing that your babies are missing the added comfort of their pacifier to soothe them back to sleep during nonfeeding wakings, you may need to go a bit slower with the Modified Shuffle process.

Dramatic Wake-Up

When you start sleep coaching, you'll want to follow Kim's 6 AM Rule: Any time a twinnie wakes before 6 AM, coach them back to sleep as you would with any night waking. For example, if one of your babies wakes at 5:30 AM, you'll coach them back to sleep until 6 AM.

However, if they are both still awake at 6 AM, then you can throw in the towel and do something Kim calls Dramatic Wake-Up to let your duo know that nighttime is officially over and it's time to start the day.

To perform Dramatic Wake-Up:

- Stand up quickly.
- Leave the room.
- Count to ten.
- Channel your inner Snow White by entering the room again happily and performing the following routine:
  — Open the blinds.
  — Say "Good morning! Nighttime is over!" in an energetic voice.
  — Pick them up and leave the sleep area.

If one twinnie does end up falling back asleep before 6 AM, you can leave them sleeping while you liberate the awake twinnie. Or, if you feel that, at 6 AM, one or both of your babies are close to falling back to sleep, feel free to coach them longer. Just make sure everyone is up for the day by 7 AM to avoid throwing off your schedule.

Your Nap Plan in Phase 2 While Sleep Coaching at Bedtime and Night Wakings

When you follow the steps for Phase 2, your sleep plan will include sleep coaching at bedtime and night wakings. As with Phase 1, the nap section of your plan will be to get naps any way you can get them while you focus on nighttime sleep coaching until you feel that your twins can be put down in their cribs for sleep time with minimal patting and shushing.

Phase 3: Nap Coaching

Deep cleansing breath. Nap coaching is often one of the most stressful parts of sleep coaching for parents. For one thing, when you're just helping your twinnies get sleep any way you can, your schedule is pretty flexible—you might be able to head out for an afternoon at the park while your babies sleep comfortably in the stroller. When you start nap coaching, you'll need to commit to being at home for the process. And sometimes it can feel like nap coaching is all that you're doing all day. But I promise, you're almost there, and the time spent on this is totally worth it! I'm excited for you just thinking about it. Having your twins on a regular schedule for eating and now sleeping is revolutionary. It's liberating and awesome. Plus, you've already come so far. I'm proud of you! Now let's do this.

Sleep Coaching at Nap Time

Typically, Kim and her team work on nap coaching with babies after they are six months old (adjusted age), so don't stress if your twins aren't ready yet.

If your babies are pros at going to sleep by themselves at night, however, you may be ready to apply the Modified Shuffle to daytime naps. Or you might choose to nap coach if the way that your babies got to sleep for naps in the past is not working now—even if you are still not "done" coaching them at night. If your twins are not sleeping well during the day, nighttime coaching can be even more of a challenge.

If you plan to nighttime coach and nap time coach concurrently, always coach first at bedtime and do your first nap coaching the following morning. Always remember, babies learn best at bedtime after a day of successful naps.

The nap coaching process is fairly similar to the one we recommend at bedtime and for night wakings. You'll start by putting your duo down in their sleep space calm but awake and then follow the same steps you used when you coached them at bedtime. However, here are a few key suggestions that apply specifically to naps:

- Start sleep coaching at the onset of the first nap of the day (which should not start before 8 AM). Your babies will have an easier time falling asleep in the morning than later on.
- At this age, your babies are probably taking three to four naps per day. Try to get your babies down for a nap in their cribs for at least two of these

naps. If you need to nap them in a stroller or a carrier for the remaining nap(s), that's just fine. Coaching at more than two naps a day can feel a bit overwhelming, and you also want to avoid your twinnies being overtired at bedtime.

- Make sure to follow your usual pre-nap time routine first, so your twins know that a nap is coming next.

- Follow the same steps you used when using the Modified Shuffle at bedtime, placing a chair next to your twins' cribs to start, but move your chair farther away every three days, even if your babies didn't nap well on the third day.

- Plan to spend around an hour coaching your babies to sleep, if needed. Use the Dramatic Wake-Up (see below) if you get to the end of the hour and they are not asleep. If an hour feels impossible, try for thirty minutes. This is the big difference between using the Modified Shuffle at nap time versus at bedtime, when we coach until they fall asleep, however long that takes. Stay in the chair and follow the guidelines for the Modified Shuffle for the time you have allotted.

- If your babies wake up before the forty-five-minute mark, or seem tired and cranky when they wake, try to coach them back to sleep. If they haven't fallen asleep after fifteen to thirty minutes, you can move to Dramatic Wake-Up.

Dramatic Wake-Up at Nap Time

When you first try nap coaching, you may find that you have been trying to get your duo to sleep for over thirty minutes. By this point, you may have a gut feeling that they just won't be going to sleep! You may also be at this point if you have tried to coach them *back* to sleep for fifteen to thirty minutes after a midnap wake-up with no success. Rather than continuing to try to get them to sleep, end the nap with Dramatic Wake-Up, the same way you would if your kiddos won't fall back to sleep in the morning before their standard morning wake time.

Dramatic Wake-Up tells your twinnies that nap time is now over. You don't want to simply stop coaching and pick them up, because they will learn to associate any fussing with being picked up. Instead, follow the directions on page 251: When you enter the room, open the blinds to let the sunshine in and say "Nap time is over!" in an energetic voice.

Your nap coaching will have four possible outcomes:

- Your babies respond well to nap coaching, go to sleep within the hour, and nap for over forty-five minutes. (Yes! Yes! Yes!)
- Your babies take only a forty-five minute nap but wake up rested. However, watch their sleepy cues (and the clock) afterward because, given this shorter nap, they may be ready for their next nap sooner.
- Your twins sleep for less than forty-five minutes. Kim calls these abbreviated naps disaster naps because your duo has not had time to go through a complete sleep cycle and will often wake cranky and tired. After a disaster nap, commit to following the Modified Shuffle steps for another fifteen to thirty minutes no matter how your twinnies respond. And as with a forty-five minutes nap, be sure to watch their sleepy cues and the clock after this because they may be ready for their next nap early.
- One or both of your duo doesn't go to sleep despite your coaching. Leave the room and perform Dramatic Wake-Up. After no sleep, their next nap will come sooner so keep your eye out for sleepy cues.

Consider first focusing on coaching for just the morning nap, then adding coaching for the second nap once you feel you are making progress with the morning nap. If you feel overwhelmed thinking about coaching the twinnies for naps during the entire day from the get-go, then don't! Successfully coaching during the morning nap can give you the win you need to feel confident moving on to the next nap.

Create Your Sleep Coaching Plan

Now it's time to devise your sleep coaching plan! I'm doing a happy dance over here for you. Sit down with your partner and twinnie helpers and make this plan together during the day. Think it through, talk it through—and write it down. Putting your plan on paper will ensure that you're all on the same page (literally and figuratively!) and help you avoid miscommunication. Most importantly, it will help you be consistent with your kiddos.

For a printable plan for you to fill out, use the QR code.

Before you begin, make sure that you can set aside three weeks to commit to your sleep coaching plan. I hope this doesn't make you roll your eyes, but I'd rather you block off too much time than not enough. Three weeks will give you plenty of nights to get through the Modified Shuffle, even if you decide to hold at one or two steps for a few extra days each.

Consider, too, what's going on in your lives. Has one of you just returned to work? Is there any extra stress you're dealing with? Changes or additional stress in your life can impact your ability to follow the sleep coaching steps consistently.

You also want to make sure your twinnie team—you, your partner, and/or any helpers—can present a united front as you sleep coach. Confirm that everyone involved in the plan is on board and that you have the support you need.

The following is a sample plan, using the template, for five-month-old twins Anna and John, who sleep in cribs.

Our Sleep Plan for: Anna and John

We met with our pediatrician and discussed any eating, growth, and general health issues we had for our twins, and we ruled out any potential underlying medical conditions that might interfere with their sleep.

Our twinnies need the following:

Total amount of nighttime sleep:	11 hours
Total amount of daytime sleep:	4 hours
Number of naps:	3, sometimes 4

After reviewing their eating and sleep logs over the last few days, we believe their natural bedtime is: 7 PM

Our daily schedule is as follows:

6 AM to 7:30 AM	Wake-up / Change / Feed
8:30 AM to 9 AM	Nap (not before 8 AM at the earliest)
10 AM to 11:30 AM	Change / Tummy time / Feed
Around noon or 1 PM	Nap
2 PM to 3 PM	Change / Tummy time / Feed
Around 3 PM or 4 PM	Nap

*Fourth nap may be needed in the early evening.

6 PM to 6:30 PM	Start bedtime routine / Feed
7 PM	Start the first step of the Modified Shuffle

Our bedtime routine will include the following:

- Bath or gentle cleaning with a washcloth.
- Massage.
- Nurse with the night-light on.
- Short song or book.
- Into crib calm but awake.

Our bedtime plan will be as follows:

- One of us will sit by one twin and the other by the other kiddo until they both fall asleep.
- We have reviewed all the rules of the Modified Shuffle.
- We will each decide when it is appropriate to pick up the twinnie we are in charge of to calm them and whether it is helping.
- We will not coach one other and will only show support. This will teach our twins what true teamwork and love look like.
- We agree that learning to put yourself to sleep is an essential life skill and the goal is to teach this to our twins.

Our positions will be as follows:

- Nights 1–3: Each parent standing/sitting by their primary baby's crib.
- Nights 4–6: Both parents or one parent sitting on a chair two feet from the cribs.

- Nights 7–9: Both parents or one parent sitting on a chair three-plus feet from the cribs (moving one foot farther away each night).

Our nighttime strategy will be as follows:

- Our pediatrician recommends the twins get one feeding during an eleven- to twelve-hour night. Currently, they are getting two.
- We will feed them at the first waking after midnight and then not until 6 AM at the earliest, and then we will start our day.
- For their first feeding, Mom will go in, change the first baby's diaper, nurse them, and place them back in the crib, then repeat the process with the other baby. (Mom will unlatch each twin once they are done with their feeding and not allow them to suckle back to sleep.)
- For their second feeding, Dad will go in, change the first baby's diaper, give them a bottle with incrementally fewer ounces over the course of three nights, put them back in their crib, and repeat the process with the other baby. On the fourth night, this second feeding will be dropped.
- If the babies are upset, one parent will go in and sit between the twins' cribs at each waking and follow the Modified Shuffle steps.
- We agree not to take the twinnies out of their room to start the day before 6 AM.
- We agree not to bring the babies into our bed.

Our nap plan will be as follows:

- We have decided not to nap coach at this time.
- We will fill the twinnies' daytime sleep tanks by getting their naps any way we can.
- We will rock them to sleep and put them to sleep in their cribs.
- If they don't fall asleep easily, we will put them in their stroller and go for a walk and let them sleep there for their nap.

Our nanny / daycare provider has agreed to the following:

Our nanny will make sure that the twins get four hours of daytime naps even if they have to sleep in the stroller or in someone's arms. We shared with her the twins' schedule and average wake window length (an hour and a half), and she is willing to work with us on the timing of their naps.

We're ready to go! We have blocked out three weeks of our schedule and are dedicating ourselves to improving our babies' sleep habits!

As you fill out your own sleep coaching plan, here are a few things to keep in mind:

1. Focus on nights first. Daytime sleep is harder and develops later, so don't fret if your twins still need help sleeping for naps (or are even still napping in their swings!).

2. Even though you're focusing on nights first, have a plan for daytime sleep. At this age, it's important to help your duo get daytime sleep any way you can. Where will your babies nap and how will you get them to sleep?

3. Review your feeding logs with your doctor and ask about your twinnies' nighttime feeding needs. How many will you include in your plan?

4. Decide how you will address night wakings and night feedings. How much nutrition did you and your pediatrician decide each twin needs at night? How will you address night wakings that are not tied to feedings? Will you be focusing on coaching at bedtime only, or at night wakings, too?

5. Take your babies' temperaments into account. How will this affect your plan?

Consistency Is Key

"Consistency Is Key" should be a tattoo all new parents get as a reminder, because this statement will ring true regardless of age when it comes to your kiddos. Consistency makes our lives easier and takes a lot of the guesswork out of our days, and sleep coaching is no different. Create your sleep plan and stick to it! With time, patience, and perseverance, the twinnies will learn the drill, and before you know it, things will fall into place.

Sleep Challenges While Sleep Coaching

No one said sleep coaching was gonna be a walk in the park. But like with many things, sometimes those that are the hardest are also the most rewarding. If you find you're running into some trouble overall, the easiest thing to do is to slow the whole process down and stay a bit longer with each step. But if you're having a specific struggle, we've got some ideas on how to fix them!

Early Rising

Have you started sleep coaching and your twins are now taking a much longer stretch at the beginning of the night, but are also waking at 4 AM or 5 AM seemingly ready to start their day? Early rising is a very common sleep struggle!

Early rising during sleep coaching is not the same as having an *early bird*—a little one who, thanks to temperament or genetics, wakes refreshed but earlier than their parents would like. Early risers are not happy when they wake at the crack of dawn. They are awake but grouchy because they didn't get enough sleep. It is a common problem because early morning is the hardest time for babies to learn to put themselves back to sleep.

The three possible causes of early rising during sleep coaching are:

1. Overtiredness at bedtime, due to a less-than-full nap tank, too long of a wake window between the last nap of the day and bedtime, or a bedtime that was too late.

2. Being put down too drowsy at bedtime (when they're put in their cribs practically asleep, they don't have the chance to master falling asleep independently, and so have more trouble at 5 AM).

3. Hunger (your babies may not quite be ready to go all night without a feeding!).

How to Help Early Risers

In order to help nip this early rising in the bud, you'll want to treat this early wake-up like any other night waking and coach your baby or babies back to sleep. If you are unable to coach them back to sleep by the time the clock strikes six, go ahead and do Dramatic Wake-Up.

Whether they get back to sleep or are up for the day, your job the next day will be to fill those daytime nap tanks. Pay attention to the length of their last wake window of the day to make sure that it's not too long. And watch their sleepy cues to make sure that they are not too overtired by bedtime.

The trick to beating early rising is to commit to coaching your twins back to sleep. Things will improve with persistence and consistency. Hang in there!

Overstimulation During Sleep Coaching

Are you worried that your twins are getting overstimulated by your presence next to them as you are putting them to sleep? This is rare, but it *can* happen. Usually, babies cry during sleep coaching from frustration: "I don't understand why you are no longer rocking me to sleep!" "I don't know how to do this on my own. Why won't you pick me up and feed me to sleep?" But sometimes a baby's crying escalates because, in an effort to soothe their babies, parents unintentionally do "too much," moving too quickly from one soothing tool to the next, and it makes their babies upset. Slow down and use the SOAR process to see which soothing tools are truly working.

Daycare and Sleep Coaching

We don't recommend that you start sleep coaching when your twins are about to start attending daycare. It's too much change at once! It's often better to wait until your baby has settled in and the new change sleep coaching represents won't be too much for them.

Even then, sleep coaching can be challenging. Some parents find that their babies don't nap well when they are at daycare (so they don't get their daytime sleep tank filled). Sometimes daycares have no nap schedule, and sometimes babies have difficulty sleeping in the daycare environment. And as you know by now, when babies don't sleep well during the day, they often don't sleep well at night. Also, some babies refuse a bottle during the day, and as a result are up more often to feed at night.

As you know, we always tell parents to start sleep coaching after a fantastic day of naps so that their babies are happy and not overtired at bedtime. If your duo hasn't been sleeping well at daycare, you may want to start sleep coaching on a Saturday night after a day of holding them for naps. You can then follow your plan, seeing if starting with two weekend days of solid napping helps jump-start the process.

We also suggest that you work with the daycare to solve napping issues. You can:

- Share your sleep coaching plan with them and see if they will work with you and your twins' needs. Share the schedule you find your twins work best with. When you drop them off each day, tell the daycare what time each of them woke and when you think they will need their next nap.
- Ask them if they are able to follow a suggested schedule.
- Have them fill your twinnies' daytime sleep tanks any way they can safely (that is, not simply letting them sleep unattended in a swing).

The goal is to have twinnies that are relatively well rested at pickup, ready to face bedtime and the night ahead.

Sleep Coaching in One Bedroom

Some families room share with their twins by choice. Others do so not because they want to, but because the size or layout of their home doesn't offer an alternative.

If you are going to start the Modified Shuffle with the twins in your room, we suggest:

- At bedtime, put your babies down in their sleep space calm but awake.
- Start by sitting next to them on your bed or in a chair.
- Follow the Modified Shuffle guidelines at bedtime (page 235).
- For wakings that occur *before* your bedtime, coach your kiddos back to sleep from your bed or chair position during the first few nights.
- At all wakings (from night 3 and on) *after* your bedtime (and *after* the time you set for a dream feed or set-time feeding, if that is part of your feeding plan), sleep coach back to sleep from your bed using verbal cues, shushing your little ones to sleep with a focus on doing less over time.

If your twinnies are sensitive to your presence in the room overnight, making it more difficult to sleep coach, and you don't have the option of moving them to a different space, you can try to minimize any disruption by placing a screen divider between their crib and your bed, using white noise to block your sounds as you move around, and having everything you need for your day in another room if you need to get up earlier than them.

Sharing a Room with a Sibling

I wouldn't recommend putting your twins in with a sibling—if at all possible—until they are sleeping through the night. It's not worth the risk of your babies waking their sibling and adding another family member to the list of those not sleeping. I was a singleton, but my mom can still remember my older sister waking up in the middle of the night to my cries, yelling, "Shut this kid up!" She's just lucky I wasn't a twin!

When to Take a Break

When you're sleep coaching, if, after thirty minutes (or even just fifteen) of the Modified Shuffle method, you're feeling like you can't take the crying or the stress of the process, you should stop. You want to be at a place where you can commit to following through. If your gut is telling you to stop, you won't be able to be consistent.

And that's OK! You can take a break. And that break can be as long or as short as you need. You could try the next day. Or you could give yourself some time to think about it and wait to start again once you are feeling like you can commit.

If you feel that the Modified Shuffle is too much, but still want to move beyond sleep shaping, you could try the Super Slow Shuffle (page 210) outlined in "Your Twins' Fourth Month." Or you can try the Jiggle and Soothe (page 173) or Jiggle and Soothe 2.0 (page 209) so that you feel you're making some progress without going full-out on sleep coaching.

Additionally, you might want to take a break when you've followed your plan for three to five nights without seeing any improvement. If you don't see things changing after three to five nights of consistent coaching, it is possible that one or both of your twins are not ready for sleep coaching (or perhaps they might even have an underlying medical condition that is making the process too difficult). You can assess the situation the next morning and decide when to start trying again.

Taking Care of You

As you're teaching your kiddos self-regulation through sleep coaching, it helps if you are also self-regulated. Because of the power of something called mirror neurons—the amazing fireworks in your twinnies' brains that cause them to match, or "mirror," what's going on in your own brain—when we are calm, it helps our babies stay calm, too.

In order for us to feel calm, we have to make sure we are taking care of ourselves—by getting enough sleep and caring for our bodies with light exercise and movement, a little meditation, or at least some deep breathing. Listen, I'll be the first to tell you that I'm the worst at this, but if I can give you just one tip from the future, it's this: You'll never regret taking a moment for yourself. It will make you a better parent, a better partner, and a better human. Please give yourself a little space to adapt. OK? For your babies. Please.

Remember, too, to trust yourself and your choices. I see so much parental guilt when well-meaning family or friends offer advice (or even judgment) about parents' sleep coaching choices. It can be difficult to hear your mom, uncle, sister, or cousin question, correct, or give unsolicited advice about how you are caring for your duo (especially if you are short on sleep and patience). During these times, it's important to remember that **you are an amazing, caring parent**. You've made the decisions you have for a reason.

If you find that your family is questioning your choice to sleep coach (especially if they are proponents of Cry It Out), don't feel the need to explain yourself. If you must explain why you are choosing to sleep coach, you can always give your family member a copy of this book or direct them to Twiniversity website (Twiniversity.com) and/or The Sleep Lady website (SleepLady.com). That way they can digest the information from a source other than you—which, for them, might lend the techniques more credibility.

You have an ally over here in me and the rest of the Twiniversity and Gentle Sleep Coach crews. No matter if it's today or fourteen years from now, we will always be here to support you in any way we can. YOU know what's best for your babies. YOU know what's best for your family. YOU know what's best for you, and no matter what that is, we support you!

FAST to Sleep Summary

Ready? Set? Sleep! You've filled your toolbox with the tools you'll need to coach your twinnies onto the Sleeptown Express! Now let's clock in and get to work on that sleep coaching plan! You got this.

What to Focus on This Month

1. Soothe your babies' stranger anxiety (page 219).
2. Feed your newly distractible eaters in a quiet room to help them avoid snacking and not eating enough during the day, which can lead to increased feedings at night.
3. If you feel like you are still recovering from the four-month sleep regression or what feels like the aftermath of it, revisit our sleep shaping tips (page 199) to get back on track.
4. Is your baby ready to start Baby-Led Sleep Coaching?
    *   Revisit the Baby-Led Sleep Coaching Readiness Checklist (page 205–206).
    *   Check with your pediatrician.
    *   Create your sleep plan (page 254), including how you will address night feedings.
    *   Decide how you will fill your twins' daytime sleep tanks.
    *   Make sure you have set aside three weeks of at-home time to focus on the sleep coaching process.
5. Find moments for yourself daily. If you don't take a break, you can burn out.

What Not to Worry About

- Forty-five-minute naps.
- Nap coaching and weaning all night feeds, if it feels like too much to take on at once (and particularly if a parent has recently started back to work).

For a printable PDF of this month's "FAST to Sleep Summary" plus helpful book bonuses, use the QR code.

Notes

chapter eight

The Most Common Twin Sleep Issues

Welcome to your *free digital chapter!* While we know that the last few hundred pages have been full of helpful tidbits on your twinnies' sleep, Kim and I both feel that nothing beats getting to see our advice in action in real-world scenarios.

In this free digital chapter, you'll find real stories from real parents, like yourself, who have sought out Kim's and my help. You'll find these families, their sleep issues, and real-life solutions in your free digital chapter:

- Megan is currently thirty-two weeks pregnant with twins. She wants to make sure that her twins will sleep their best after delivery and is looking for advice on one crib or two and if they should sleep in her room or in their own nursery.
- Ben and Alex were born at thirty-four weeks and are one month old. They both have very bad reflux and their parents are worried they aren't getting enough sleep.
- Charlotte and Nora were born at thirty-five and a half weeks and are two months old. They have no real schedule and have been feeding and sleeping on demand. It's been a rough eight weeks for their parents, who would like to get Charlotte's and Nora's sleeping more organized but don't know how to start.

- Emily and Abigale were born at thirty-three weeks and are three months old. They sleep great during the day but get up almost hourly overnight. Dad works overnights and Mom is flying solo and needs guidance on how to do this alone.
- Miguel and Eva were born at thirty-eight weeks and are three months old. Miguel has colic and doesn't sleep through the night. He seems exhausted all day. Eva is a great sleeper for naps and overnight. They are wondering if they should have them sleep in separate rooms so Miguel doesn't wake Eva up.
- Miles and Lucy were born at thirty-five weeks and are four months old. Their parents are still rocking them to sleep with a bottle. Even when they wake up in the middle of the night, they need to be rocked to sleep. The parents are at their wits' end, utterly exhausted, and looking for sleep help.
- Fredrick and Isabella were born at thirty-eight weeks and are five months old. Mom is returning to work soon and plans to put them in preschool. They don't do well for naps, and overnights aren't great, either. They still get a 3 AM bottle. Mom worries about getting up overnight when she needs to be at her best during the day.

However, since this *is* a digital chapter, we are able to update it with questions and answers pretty often. Drop by to see what new families we've included!

Twin sleep issues are really, really common. At Twiniversity, we remind parents that raising twins isn't just twice as hard—it's honestly exponentially more challenging—but it's also exponentially more rewarding. We are here to help you every step of the way. Remember we have classes and—what our families have found they need most—monthly virtual meetups where you can join us on video from around the world and share your twin sleep challenges, and collectively, as a community, we'll try to come up with a realistic solution. You can also take a Twiniversity class or book a session with Kim, her coaches, or even little old me. Just use the QR code at the start of this chapter to find the links. We are excited to help you get your twinnies sleeping through the night—but more importantly, we are excited to help *you* sleep through the night, too.

chapter nine

What's Next?

Holy moly guacamole! I'm so freaking proud of you guys. You did it! You got to this point, and I'm praying that your brains aren't spilling out of your ears with all that you've learned over the last (what feels like) ten million pages.

If your babies are already here, I'm hoping that by the time you get to this final chapter, you'll be well rested and that all the tips worked the way they should (though you know what they say about "should"—see page 24).

If you picked up this book during your pregnancy, I hope you've learned how to take the sleep coaching process step-by-step and now have more realistic expectations on what to expect.

Over the next several months, whenever you decide to go all in on sleep coaching, give your family and friends the heads-up. Tell them that you are ready to teach your babies their next skill, and that's how to soothe themselves. Tell them what kind of support you'd like from them, whether it's prepping some freezer meals, a standing commitment to mow your lawn, or even help with sleep coaching itself. We've had plenty of grandmas and grandpas of twins roll their sleeves up when it comes to sleep coaching, so maybe even share your copy of this book with them or get them a copy of their own. The famous saying is "It takes a village"—welcome with open arms anyone you trust who wants to be part of your twin village.

Once my twins were on a good sleep and feeding schedule, I guarded it like it was a mine full of gold. I didn't deviate much, and I have no regrets about it. I'll admit it, I missed some holidays and special occasions, but knowing they would fall asleep soundly each night at 7:30 was my salvation. The first year was FULL of ups and downs, and my twins' daily schedule was the consistency I needed to feel like a human. It's OK to say no to some things. Be picky about where you go and who you're with at this stage of your twins' lives. They will only be this little once; it's a very temporary time in life, so make the choices you feel are best for the team.

Now, maybe you've gotten to this page and things haven't gone as planned. Maybe the process was harder than you expected, or maybe your doc said your twinnies still need plenty of feeds overnight. It's OK! We can pick up and try again. A lot of our kiddos are born early. Heck, I've worked with more twenty-nine-weekers this year than I have in the past decade. Everyone is on their own timeline—especially when you have two. My own babies, born at thirty-four weeks, had a lot of sleep struggles, and it took me a lot more time to realize the importance of adjusted age than I care to admit. In truth, there are a lot of reasons you might need to change your exact plans when your twins are under six months. That's why I push you to speak to your doctor often. Us twin parents, we have to. But even if you had a singleton born at forty weeks, I'd still tell you to get the OK to sleep train from your doc.

If you're here and still need more help, lean on us. Kim and her Gentle Sleep Coaches are specifically trained to work with multiple-birth families. I've worked with many of them personally, so I know they will help you so, so much. Don't be afraid to reach out to them—or to me, either. Visit Twiniversity.com/gentlesleep to find someone near you.

Sweet dreams,
Nat

Acknowledgments

Is it weird that when I read a book, I always go to the acknowledgments section first? I feel like it gives me a sense of the author, and if the acknowledgments are good, I enjoy the book more. Yeah. I'm a weirdo. So here are mine, and I'm totally cool if you read this first.

(Clears throat and hold up glass to make a toast.) Who knew that 712 years ago, when I met Ms. Kim West, that my name would be sitting next to hers on the cover of a book? I didn't. Kim, from the moment we met and you instantly jumped into a random ball pit with me in Los Angeles, I knew you were my kind of person! You're amazing. I joke with you a lot, but seriously, I'm in awe of your knowledge and passion regarding not only pediatric sleep but also life, motherhood, entrepreneurship, and continuous learning. Sincerely, thank you for sharing your immense knowledge with me and allowing me to share your world of Gentle Sleep Coaching with my peeps. I know that you and I made beautiful music together on these pages, and I look forward to our next project, even if it's just a few drinks on a balcony. But for real, I'm never going to a sushi restaurant with you again. So, raise your glass. Cheers to the amazing Kim West. (Roaring applause.)

(Reader, I'll let you in on the sushi situation. I was with Kim in New York City where I ended up getting the most horrific food poisoning of my life. I'm still traumatized more than a decade later.)

I also want to thank Leah Wilson and the BenBella team for their enormous amount of patience with me and for helping Kim and me get this book off the ground in less than a year. Leah, toward the end of the whole editing process, I literally couldn't tell what you edited and what I wrote. You're amazing. My favorite note: "It needs a little more Nat here." You rock my world, missy!

Thank you to my Twiniversity team for holding down the fort so I could focus on the pages you're holding in your hands now. I never imagined that I could find a group of women as dedicated as I am to making the lives of twin families better. You guys are amazing, and I humbly thank you!

Babe. Thank you for allowing my "hobby" to grow and for supporting (and pushing) me through it all. Hey, listen, without you, Alexa would never know the word *Twiniversity*. You're something else, my love, and I can't wait to read your acknowledgments when you're ready.

Twinnies, you're all grown up, but you will always be my babies. I'm amazed how the tables have turned and you guys are constantly encouraging ME. Anna, I'm not letting my dreams be dreams, look at that! And John, I'm not giving all my advice away for free. I love how you look out for me. You two are my everything, and if there was only one of you . . . ahhh, that would be tough, but you know who my favorite is. (Psst. It's you. Don't tell your twin.)

Hey, Ma! Thank you. Your cups of tea and random lunches gave me the energy to put my fingers on this keyboard most days. And no, I'm not paying you for your services.

Trixie, Auntie, Francini, Rog, Bag of D girls, and the rest of the gang of misfit toys that love me, if it wasn't for the (insert what you've done for me lately while I was struggling to get this book done), I don't know if I would have made it to my final word.

And one more thing, thank you to every single person buying this book. If you're buying it for yourself or as a gift, or just looted it to use as toilet paper when the apocalypse arrived, thank you. Thank you for validating the need for more twin-specific information in this world and for allowing me to be a spokesperson on behalf of our twinning community since 2009. Thank you for taking our classes, listening to our podcast, buying our app, and coming day in and day out to our website. You guys gave my life a purpose that I did not anticipate. I'm humbled by all the support you continuously give Twiniversity, and I look forward to supporting even more generations of new families of twins. Thank you.

—Nat

It's true Nat and I hit it off from the first time we were thrown on a stage together. And yes, we could have just stayed friends (because, let me tell you, Nat is a deeply loyal, caring, and protective friend, and just the right person to call when you need a good laugh!), but her commitment, compassion, and love for her twin community has kept us forever connected in our mission to support and empower parents. Thank you, Nat, for loving and supporting me and my daughters, and most of all for teaching me and deepening my understanding of life with twins. Thank you for saying YES to coauthoring this book with me. Friends for life!

Thank you, Leah and the BenBella team, for seeing our vision . . . that parents of twins need their own book and not just a book about singletons that they have to "figure out" how to apply to their twins while feeling largely misunderstood during the process!

I had always wanted to be a parent of twins—one pregnancy two babies sounded perfect (and I would have totally been a groupie of Twiniversity and my beloved Nat)—but alas, that was not what I was given. I have worked with the parents of thousands of twins, quite a few triplets, and one set of quadruplets, and through those experiences, I learned what I *really* love about your community or tribe. You are patient and supportive of each other. You understand how much harder it is to parent multiples and aren't quick to judge or criticize each other. You have a unique and special tribe.

Although parenthood may feel unbearably hard right now, you are a forever member of an exclusive parenting club where just a look from another parent of twins brings you automatic understanding, empathy, and support. Soak it up!

I am honored to have been trusted by many of you over the years and now to have you allow Nat and me to help you navigate these first five months. Big hugs!

—Kim, The Sleep Lady

Index

A

AAP (American Academy of Pediatrics).
  See American Academy of
  Pediatrics
active sleep (REM Sleep), 89, 182
active/fussy babies. *See* alert babies
adults. *See also* parents
  number needed, 6
age. *See* fifth month; fourth month;
  newborns; second month; third
  month
age, adjusted, 16, 43, 99, 270
alert babies, 84–86, 132, 196. *See also*
  temperament
  cues of, 164
  kangaroo care and, 133
  massage and, 133
  naps and, 133
  newborns, 85–86
  sensory sensitivities and, 132
  sleep and, 162–165, 230
  sleep coaching and, 163, 197,
    230–231, 233
  sleep environment/area and, 133
  sleep shaping and, 163
  sleep strategies and, 197
  soothing and, 197

supporting, 132
touch and, 133
zone system, 132
allergies, 60, 161
American Academy of Pediatrics (AAP),
  34–35, 62, 221
  on feeding schedules, 54
  on pacifiers, 77
  on solids, 222
anxiety, 22, 29, 103, 104. *See also*
  perinatal mood and anxiety
  disorders (PMAD)
  parents', 24
Assess. *See* Stop, Observe, Assess,
  Respond (SOAR)
assistance, outside, 27–28
attachment, 11, 12, 45, 71, 134, 229.
  See also bonding; soothing
  before birth, 21–22
  bonding and, 65
  during fifth month, 225
  during first month, 64–71
  during fourth month, 189
  schedules/routines and, 160
  during second month, 122–123
  during third month, 160
attachment parenting, 64–65

About the Authors

Natalie Diaz, the "Big Cheese" over at Twiniversity (that's her official title), has been the Pied Piper of twin families since 2009. Natalie has single-handedly changed the way expecting and new parents of twins operate. A twin parent herself, Natalie has made twin parenting information mainstream with her best-selling book *What to Do When You're Having Two*, her award-winning website Twiniversity.com, the most inclusive twin parenting app on the market, her extraordinary podcasts, and creative and educational classes about all things twins. Today, she's reaching over two million families a week with Twiniversity's nurturing and supportive environment created just for twin families.

Natalie is also a twin-specific lactation professional, a child passenger safety technician, and a trained childbirth educator. She's received numerous accolades within the baby and parenting industry and has been featured in major worldwide publications and on national television helping the world have a better experience with their own twin parenting adventure.

Kim West, MSW, is a mom of two who has been a practicing child and family social worker for over twenty-five years. She has personally helped over twenty thousand families all over the world gently teach their children how to fall asleep—and fall back asleep—without leaving them to cry it out alone. She started training Gentle Sleep Coaches internationally in 2010 and has appeared as a child sleep expert in numerous magazines, newspapers, and on television programs including *Dr. Phil*, *Today*, and *Good Morning America*.

ALSO BY NATALIE DIAZ

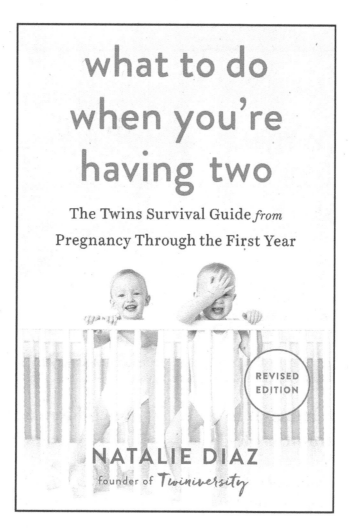

Funny, reassuring, and full of stories and advice from Natalie Diaz and other twin moms, *What to Do When You're Having Two* provides a no-holds-barred resource about life with twins, from pregnancy and birth all the way through your duo's first year of life.

Available everywhere books are sold.

FOR MORE RESOURCES, CLASSES, AND TIPS, VISIT TWINIVERSITY.COM

MORE SLEEP SUPPORT

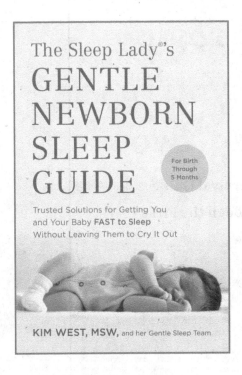

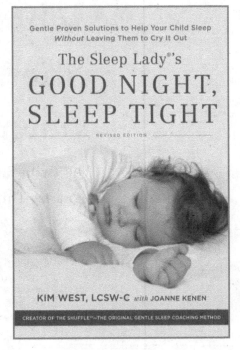

For babies 0 to 5 months old	For children 6 months to 6 years old
Outlines baby-led sleep shaping and coaching^{SM}	*Outlines The Sleep Lady Shuffle*^{SM}
A gentle approach that parents can use to first shape their baby's sleep and then, when developmentally appropriate (and according to their baby's unique temperament), coach their little one as they learn to fall asleep and stay asleep on their own	A gentle sleep coaching method that does not involve leaving your child to cry it out alone

Available everywhere books are sold.

FROM KIM WEST, THE SLEEP LADY®

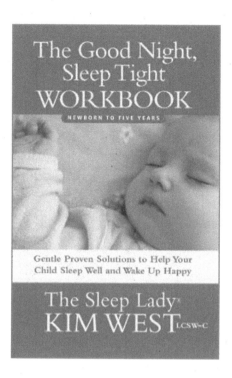

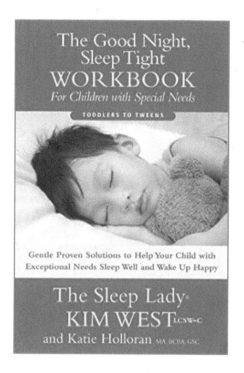

For children 0 months to 5 years old

Companion workbook to
The Sleep Lady's Good Night, Sleep Tight

A step-by-step guide, including lists, plans and logs to help tired parents with children of any age who are experiencing sleep problems

For toddlers to tweens with exceptional needs

Companion workbook to
The Sleep Lady's Good Night, Sleep Tight

Helps tired parents create and follow an effective sleep plan to achieve sleep success for their kids with special needs

FOR MORE RESOURCES, CLASSES, AND TIPS, VISIT SLEEPLADY.COM